The Basic Provider

Assisting with Advanced Life Support Skills

MW01553763

The Basic Provider

Assisting with Advanced Life Support Skills

Orlando J. Dominguez, Jr., BS, EMT-P

EMS and Critical Care Education Program Director
Health First Training Center/Brevard County Fire Rescue
Melbourne, Florida

Dr. John R. McPherson, MD, FACEP

Chair, Emergency Department
Palm Bay Community Hospital and Holmes Regional Medical Center
East Central, Florida
Medical Director, Brevard County Fire and Rescue
Melbourne, Florida

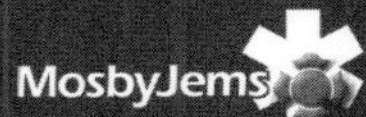

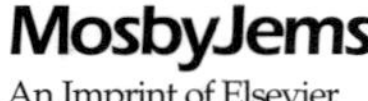

MosbyJems

An Imprint of Elsevier

THE BASIC PROVIDER
ASSISTING WITH ADVANCED LIFE SUPPORT SKILLS   0-323-02231-6
Copyright © 2004, Mosby, Inc. All right reserved

No part of this publication may be reproduced, stored in a retrieval system, or transmitted in any form or by any means, electronic, mechanical, photocopying, recording, or otherwise, without prior permission of the publisher.

NOTICE

EMS is an ever-changing field. Standard safety precautions must be followed, but as new research and clinical experience broaden our knowledge, changes in treatment and drug therapy may become necessary or appropriate. Readers are advised to check the most current product information provided by the manufacturer of each drug to be administered to verify the recommended dose, the method and duration of administration, and contraindications. It is the responsibility of the licensed prescriber, relying on experience and knowledge of the patient, to determine dosages and the best treatment for each individual patient. Neither the publisher nor the editor assumes any liability for any injury and/or damage to persons or property arising from this publication.

International Standard Book Number 0-323-02231-6

Publishing Director: Andrew Allen
Associate Developmental Editor: Kristin Armstrong
Senior Developmental Editor: Kelly Trakalo
Publishing Services Manager: Peggy Fagen
Designer: Mark Bernard

Printed in Mexico

Last digit is the print number: 9 8 7 6 5 4 3 2 1

Preface

The Basic Provider: Assisting with Advanced Life Support Skills enhances the knowledge of all basic level prehospital care providers and promotes teamwork between basic and advanced providers when caring for ill or injured patients. During an emergency, time is of the essence. Advanced providers cannot instruct basic providers on how to help with advanced skills during an advanced life support (ALS) scenario. Taking the time to learn these skills before the emergency helps avoid delays in future patient care. **This text does not promote the initiation of advanced medical procedures to be carried out by the basic provider without training and medical oversight.** Nevertheless, if you work with advanced providers in the prehospital setting, if you are assigned to an engine company that responds to medical emergencies, or if you assist in the emergency department, then this text is for you.

Although many procedures become familiar as the basic provider assists the advanced provider, five steps often need to be taken before or during transport to the hospital for every patient who requires ALS interventions: (1) oxygen administration, (2) intravenous line, (3) pulse oximeter application, (4) electrocardiographic (ECG) application, and (5) glucose check, depending on your local protocols. Completing these five steps will help you anticipate the needs of the advanced provider and will generally need to be taken to enable the advanced provider to record a baseline and to move to more definitive ALS treatments. These steps are referred to as **ALS Passport** within this text.

A companion CD-ROM is enclosed and includes videotape clips of actual procedures and reviews the techniques discussed in this text.

In addition to the text and CD-ROM, *The Basic Provider: Assisting with Advanced Life Support Skills* is also available as a continuing education course. This course is made up of both didactic information and practical skill application. The basic provider is introduced to the more common medical emergencies encountered in the prehospital setting and the appropriate ALS interventions. The basic provider has then an opportunity for hands-on application during the practical portion of the program. The course familiarizes the basic provider with advanced medical information and with the different types of equipment used during an ALS scenario. Many basic providers have complimented the course because of its nonstressful and easy-to-follow format. For more information about the course, contact your MosbyJems sales representative, or visit http://evolve.elsevier.com/Dominguez.

The objectives of *The Basic Provider: Assisting with Advanced Life Support Skills*, the CD-ROM, the instructional materials, and the course are to:

1. Promote teamwork between basic and advanced providers.
2. Familiarize the first responder and basic provider with ALS equipment.
3. Review medical emergencies and their treatments in the emergency ALS setting.
4. Discuss situations during which advanced skills might be needed.

I hope this text is the beginning of a new trend in emergency medical services (EMS). It is through continuous training, planning, and hands-on application that the basic provider can truly use the skills authorized by their advanced provider teammates to their fullest, helping the advanced providers deliver timely ALS care. As long as all prehospital care providers continue to work together, EMS will always be an example of dedicated medical professionals.

Orlando J. Dominguez, Jr., BS, EMT-P
John R. McPherson, MD, FACEP

Author Acknowledgments

I would like to first thank God for blessing me with such a wonderful opportunity. In addition, I would like to thank Jennifer, "My Little Bear," for all her hugs and patience while daddy was working on this project. Many thanks are also extended to my mother for her encouragement and for believing in me. Last, thanks to Claire Merrick, Kelly Trakalo, Kristin Armstrong, and Dr. McPherson, and to all those who assisted me in making a dream come true.

Orlando J. Dominguez, Jr.

Publisher Acknowledgments

The editors wish to acknowledge and thank the following reviewers. Their comments were enlightening and invaluable in helping develop this first edition.

John Doty, EMT
EMS Coordinator
Brevard County Fire Rescue
Rockledge, Florida

Kenneth Jarrett, EMT-P
Field Training Officer
American Medical Response
San Antonio, Texas

Michael Lynch, NREMT-P,
 CCEMT-P
Administrative Director
Crozer Chester Medical Center
Emergency Medical Services
 Training Institute
Upland, Pennsylvania

David Pecora, MS, PA-C,
 NREMT-P
Chief, Physician Assistant/
 Clinical Instructor
West Virginia University,
 Department of Emergency
 Medicine
Morgantown, West Virginia

Paul Phrampus, MD
Assistant Professor of
 Emergency Medicine
University of Pittsburgh
Pittsburgh, Pennsylvania

Scott Seppelt, EMT-B
Deputy Chief
Florissant Fire District
Florissant, Missouri

Debra LeJeune, MEd,
 NREMT-P
Instructor and Education
 Coordinator
Emergency Medicine
 Program
University of Pittsburgh,
Pittsburgh, Pennsylvania

We would like to give a special thanks to Debra LeJeune for her work on the procedure skills in the companion CD-ROM and her overall advice on the project.

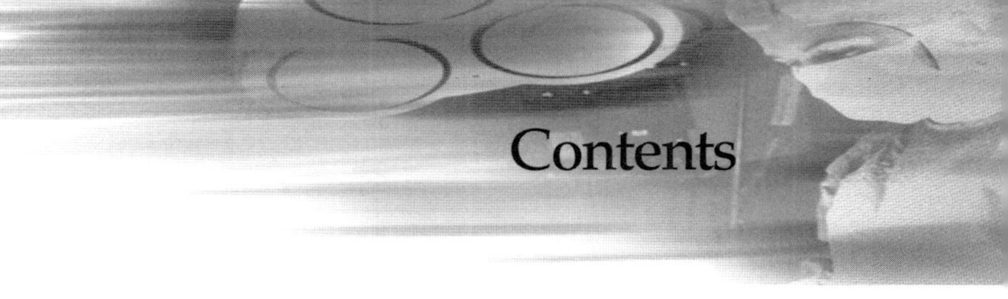

Contents

ALS Conditions Requiring BLS Procedures

Anatomy and Physiology Review

CHAPTER 1

Objectives

After completing this chapter, you will be able to:
1. *Define the listed key terms.*
2. *Identify the components of the upper and lower airways.*
3. *Explain the mechanics of the respiratory system.*
4. *Explain how respiratory gases diffuse.*
5. *Explain the flow of blood through the heart.*
6. *Differentiate depolarization and repolarization.*
7. *List the functions of the sinoatrial and atrioventricular nodes.*
8. *Identify the function of the Purkinje fibers.*

Key Terms

Aortic semilunar valve *Determines the outflow of blood from the left ventricle. It is located at the exit point of the left ventricle, where it opens into the aorta.*

Atria *Upper chambers of the heart.*

Atrioventricular node *Specialized cells located in the lower portion of the right atrium that allows electrical impulses from the sinoatrial node to travel into the ventricles.*

Bicuspid or mitral valve *Valve located between the left atrium and left ventricle.*

Bronchioles *Small tubes that branch off the left or right bronchus and lead to the alveolar sacs.*

Carina *Point at which the trachea divides into the right and left bronchi.*

Chemoreceptors *Sensory nerve cells located in the carotid arteries and aortic arch, which detect changes in oxygen, carbon dioxide, and pH levels.*

Coronary arteries *Responsible for supplying the heart with oxygen and nutrients. The left coronary artery is typically referred to as the "widow maker" because severe proximal occlusion of this vessel prevents blood flow to both the left anterior descending and the left circumflex artery (branches of the left coronary artery). Death would often be imminent.*

Pulmonary semilunar valve *Determines the outflow of blood from the right ventricle. It is located at the exit point of the right ventricle, where it opens into the pulmonary arteries.*

Purkinje fibers *Elaborate web of specialized electrically conducting fibers that extend through the bundle of His and bundle branches throughout the myocardial tissue for the purpose of propagating electrical impulses to the muscle to cause contraction of the heart.*

Sinoatrial node *Normal pacemaker of the heart that typically fires at a rate between 60 and 100 beats per minute in adults.*

Tricuspid valve *Valve between the right atrium and right ventricle.*

Ventricles *Lower chambers of the heart.*

RESPIRATORY SYSTEM

The respiratory system serves two major functions: it adds oxygen to the blood and it removes carbon dioxide from the blood (Figure 1-1). Oxygen is necessary to sustain life, and carbon dioxide is the by-product of cell metabolism. An interruption in the supply of oxygen or the removal of carbon dioxide can lead to shock and death.

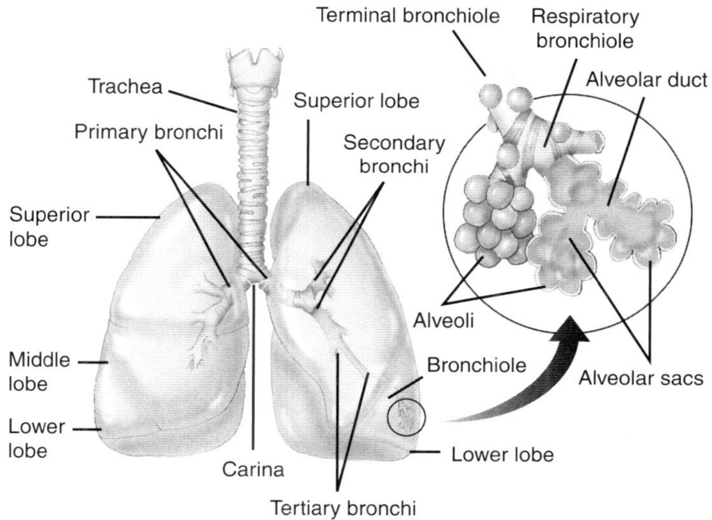

Figure 1-1 Respiratory system.

Various reflexes, nerve, and chemical responses in different locations of the body control respiration. The primary neurologic respiratory center is located in the brainstem. Respiration is also controlled by central and peripheral chemoreceptors located at the junction of the external and internal carotid arteries and the aorta. Once air is inhaled through the mouth or nose, it travels through the glottic opening and enters the trachea. The trachea divides at the carina into the right and left mainstem bronchi. The air travels through the bronchioles and then enters the alveolar sacs, which are found at the distal end of the bronchioles. Diffusion takes place at the alveoli. Diffusion is the process in which particles in fluid or gas move from an area of high concentration to an area of low concentration, resulting in an even distribution of particles in the fluid or gas. A network of pulmonary capillaries surrounds the alveolar sacs to form the alveolar-capillary membrane. The pulmonary capillaries are in close proximity to the alveolar sacs, and it is through the thin cell walls that diffusion occurs. Oxygen diffuses across the alveolar membrane into the blood within the pulmonary capillaries where the concentration of oxygen becomes lower. To be eliminated on exhalation, carbon dioxide diffuses from the blood into the alveolar sacs.

If any disruption in the respiratory system occurs, inadequate diffusion of gases may result, leading to inadequate level of oxygen or too much carbon dioxide. Such disruptions include (1) hypoventilation, (2) low oxygen environments, (3) fluid in the alveoli, (4) hypovolemia, (5) low red blood cell count or anemia, or (6) disruption or thickening of the alveolar-capillary interface.

CARDIOVASCULAR SYSTEM

The cardiovascular system consists of a pump (heart), pipes (vessels), and fluid (blood) (Figure 1-2). The heart is a muscular organ that is divided into four chambers: the right and left atria and the right and left ventricles. The right side of the heart collects deoxygenated blood, and the left side collects and delivers oxygenated blood. The deoxygenated blood reaches the heart through the inferior and superior venae cavae, which brings blood from the body to the right atrium. Once the blood reaches the heart, the right and left atria begin to fill. When both atria are filled, they contract, and the tricuspid valve and bicuspid or mitral valve open, and blood is ejected into the right and left ventricles. The ventricles then fill with blood; once filled, both ventricles contract and eject blood. The right ventricle ejects blood through the pulmonic semilunar valve into the lungs. The blood reaches the lungs through the pulmonary artery. Blood picks up oxygen and releases carbon dioxide at the lungs, which is then exhaled through the respiratory tract into the atmosphere. The oxygenated blood then returns to the left atrium. The left atrium fills, and the blood is ejected into the left ventricle. The left ventricle contracts and ejects

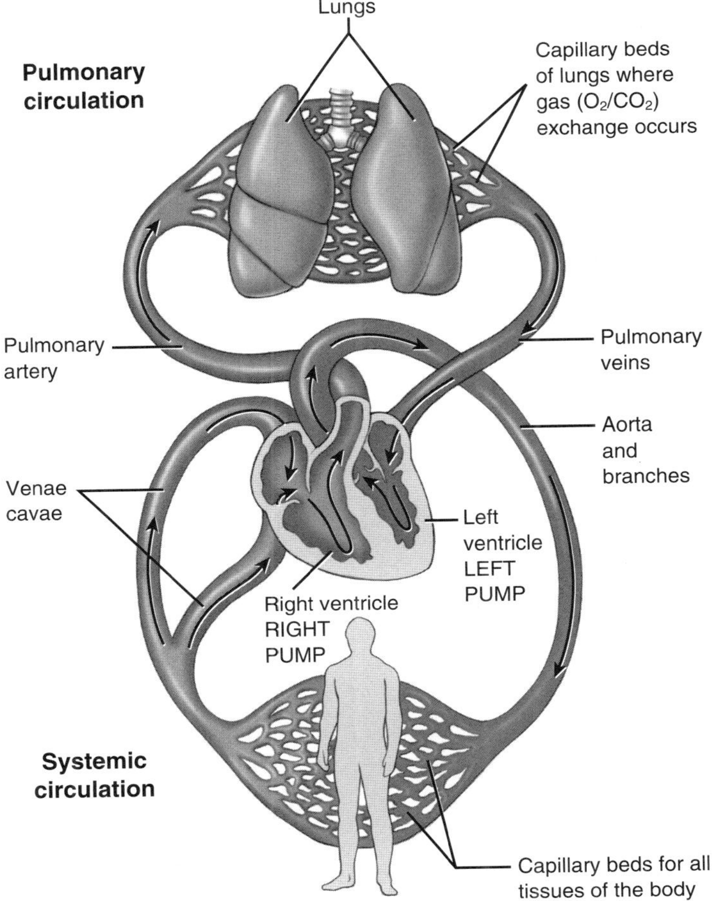

Figure 1-2 Cardiovascular system.

blood through the aortic semilunar valve into the aorta, which then transports oxygenated blood to the body as the aorta branches into other major arteries.

In addition to mechanical properties, such as pumping action, the heart also has electrical properties. For the heart to contract, it must first be stimulated to contract. The entire heart muscle has myocardial cells that respond to an electrical stimulus that causes the heart muscle to contract. How are the cells stimulated? All healthy hearts have specific sites called *pacemaker sites.* For example, the main pacemaker site is located in the right atrium of the heart. This site is called the sinoatrial node or SA node for short. What does the SA node do? It initiates the stimulus. As this electrical impulse travels down toward the ventricles via several pathways, cardiac muscle cells in the atria contract. Blood is then ejected from the atria into the ventricles. When the impulse reaches the ventricles, the ventricular cardiac muscle cells are stimulated to contract, ejecting blood from both ventricles. The blood then leaves the right ventricle for the lungs to pick up fresh oxygenated blood and deliver carbon dioxide into the alveolar sacs. The blood then returns to the left side of the heart (oxygenated side), first into the left atrium and then into the left ventricle. The blood that leaves the left ventricle exits through the aorta into the body and into the coronary arteries to feed the heart.

Stimulation of myocardial cells is referred to as *depolarization.* After the cells have been depolarized, they return to their normal resting state. This state is called *repolarization.* In addition to the SA node, several other sites have pacemaking capabilities. For example, an area called the atrioventricular (AV) node is located between the atria and the ventricles; it can also generate an electrical impulse. Additionally, the Purkinje fibers in the ventricles can generate their own impulses, causing the ventricles to depolarize. It is important to remember that depolarization does not necessarily represent contraction.

Airway

Objectives

After completing this chapter, you will be able to:
1. *Define the listed key terms.*
2. *Explain the purpose of endotracheal intubation.*
3. *Explain the purpose of endotracheal suctioning.*
4. *Explain the purpose of chest decompression.*
5. *Identify the medications that can be administered through the endotracheal route.*
6. *Identify a patient's airway needs and how to assist advanced providers.*

Key Terms

Cricoid pressure *Pressure applied over the cricoid cartilage to reduce the possibility of regurgitation and therefore aspiration by occluding the esophagus during airway maneuvers. This maneuver may also be referred to as Sellick's maneuver and is critically important when managing the airway of a patient who has already increased gastric distention as a result of bag-valve-mask ventilation.*

Endotracheal tube *Plastic tube that is placed in the trachea to provide an airway.*

End-tidal carbon dioxide detector *Sensor device attached to an endotracheal tube that detects the presence of carbon dioxide in exhaled air.*

Epigastrium *Upper region of the stomach.*

Gag reflex *Response to stimulation of the upper palate or posterior oropharynx, causing many individuals to gag or vomit or both.*

Laryngoscope *Instrument that consists of a handle and blade. It is used for examining the larynx and for assisting in the completion of procedures related to airway and pulmonary maintenance, such as foreign body removal and endotracheal intubation.*

Larynx (voice box) *Organ in the neck that consists of the thyroid cartilage, cricoid cartilage, and vocal cords. The larynx has three important functions: (1) control of airflow during breathing, (2) protection of the airway, and (3) production of sound for speech.*

Magill forceps *Elongated pair of forceps used to advance an endotracheal tube during intubation or to remove a foreign body during complete airway obstruction.*

Nasotracheal intubation *Placement of an endotracheal tube into the trachea through the nose.*

Orotracheal intubation *Placement of an endotracheal tube into the trachea through the oral cavity.*

Pulse oximeter *Device that indirectly measures the saturation of oxygen in the hemoglobin contained in red blood cells.*

Sellick's maneuver See Cricoid pressure.

Stylet *Metal probe or rod that passes through a catheter, needle, or tube. This device is used to stiffen an otherwise flexible tool to facilitate insertion. A stylet is inserted to form the endotracheal tube and is removed after orotracheal intubation.*

Vocal cords *Most important part of the larynx made of muscle and cartilage. It is covered with a thick layer of mucosa, which is critical for the production of sound for speech and for appropriately opening and closing the airway for breathing and swallowing.*

INTRODUCTION

Airway management is an essential component of prehospital medicine and of the advanced life support (ALS) Passport (see below). The advanced provider who has had hours of skill training performs the following advanced airway procedures. This chapter is designed to help the basic provider become familiar with these advanced airway procedures and to provide hints on how to assist an advanced provider during emergency airway situations.

> Remember that the ALS Passport generally consists of the five essential components that need to be carried out on all unstable or potentially unstable patients before or during transport to the hospital: (1) oxygen administration, (2) intravenous (IV) line, (3) pulse oximetry, (4) electrocardiographic (ECG) application, and (5) glucose check (depending on your local protocols).

ADVANCED LIFE SUPPORT FOR BASIC LIFE SUPPORT PROCEDURES

ENDOTRACHEAL INTUBATION

Endotracheal (ET) intubation is the insertion of a tube into the trachea. This procedure is usually accomplished by orotracheal intubation (passing a plastic tube through the mouth) or nasotracheal intubation (through the nose). The primary purpose of intubation is to establish and maintain the airway for adequate ventilation and oxygenation. Intubation requires a high degree of skill and is usually completed by advanced level providers.

Advantages:

- Provides 100% oxygen
- Prevents gastric distention
- Prevents aspiration
- Allows administration of some medications:
    1. naloxone (Narcan)
    2. epinephrine
    3. atropine
    4. lidocaine
- Allows for tracheal suctioning

OROTRACHEAL INTUBATION

Orotracheal intubation is the most common type of intubation performed in the field. The companion CD-ROM to this text provides additional information on orotracheal intubation.

When will I see it?

- Patient has severe respiratory distress.
- Patient has apnea (not breathing).
- Risk of aspiration is present (the patient has no gag reflex and is unable to protect the airway).
- Patient cannot be ventilated with other airway adjuncts.

When won't I see it?

- No respiratory distress is present.
- Patient is able to protect his or her airway from aspiration.
- Patient can be well ventilated with other airway adjuncts.

What should I watch for?

- Fluid or solid matter in the airway may hamper orotracheal intubation; therefore suction equipment should be immediately available.

- An intubation attempt should not take more than 20 seconds. After 20 seconds without successful intubation, the patient should be ventilated or oxygenated by bag-valve-mask (BVM) resuscitator before an additional attempt.
- The prehospital care team should ensure that the ET tube has been properly inserted into the trachea and not the esophagus by standard tube placement verification methods described later in the text.

Equipment

- *10 mL syringe.* The syringe is used to inflate the cuff at the distal portion of the ET tube after insertion into the trachea. The pilot balloon at the proximal portion of the ET tube will inflate as air is inserted.
- *BVM resuscitator.*
- *ET tubes.* Tubes come in a range of sizes up to 9.0 mm. The numbers represent the internal diameter of the tube. ET tubes 6.0 mm and larger have a cuff at the distal end of the tube (Figure 2-1). The average woman requires a tube measuring 7.0 to 8.0 mm, and 7.5 to 8.5 mm is the size

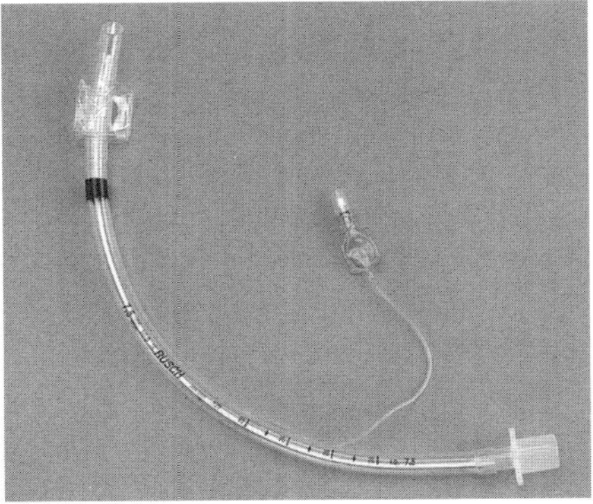

Figure 2-1 Endotracheal tube.

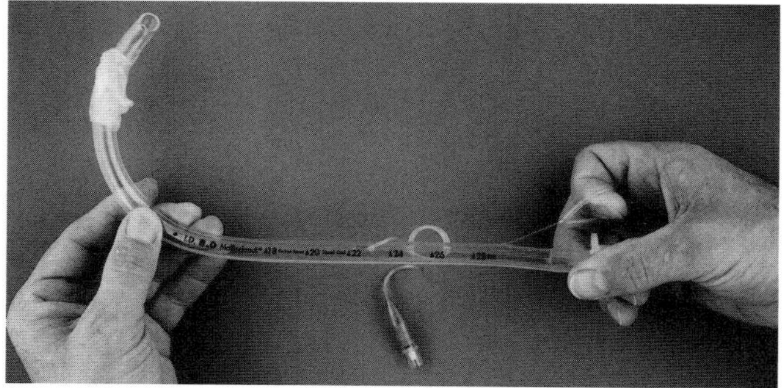

Figure 2-2 Endotrol (trigger) tube has a string. When pulled, it directs the tip anteriorly during intubation attempts.

generally used for the average man. Measuring the tube's diameter with the tip of the patient's little finger or by the diameter of the patient's nares can help determine the size to use. Length-based tapes for pediatric emergency medical dosing and appropriate equipment size should be used to assess pediatric needs.

- ▸ Children under 8 years of age do not require a cuffed tube. In the pediatric age group, the narrowest portion of the trachea is the cricoid region. If a cuffed tube is used and the cuff is inflated, it may rupture the trachea.
- ▸ Trigger tubes, also known as Endotrol tubes, provide good manual curvature of the tube throughout nasotracheal insertion, thus improving the likelihood of successful intubation in patients with a more anterior larynx (greater curvature from the posterior pharynx to the larynx) (Figure 2-2).

- *ET tube holder.* The prehospital care provider may use a commercial ET tube holder. Medical tape also may be used to secure the ET tube.
- *End-tidal carbon dioxide detector.* The end-tidal carbon dioxide detector is used to confirm the patient's expiratory carbon dioxide, which is represented by a yellow color change on

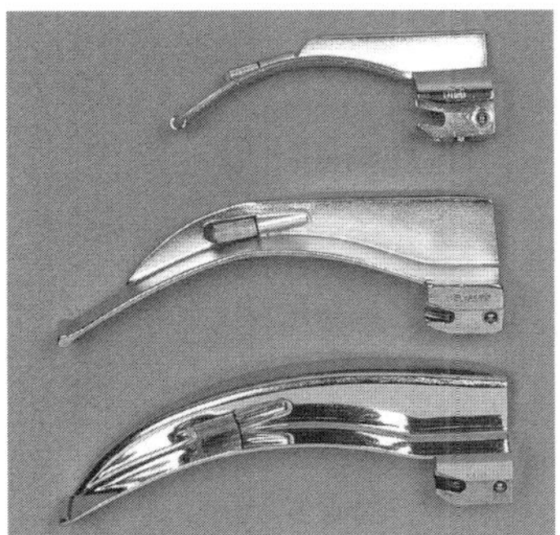

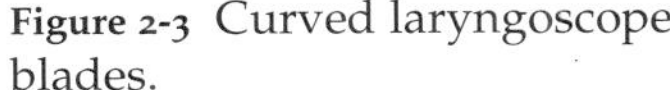

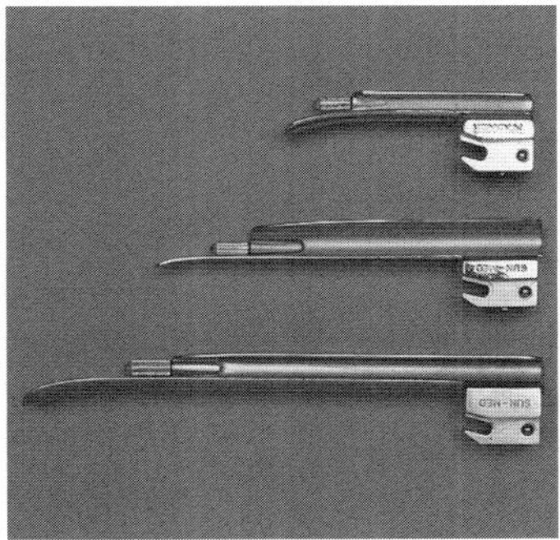

Figure 2-3 Curved laryngoscope blades.

Figure 2-4 Straight laryngoscope blades.

the litmus paper in the carbon dioxide detector. If the color in the detector is yellow after at least six ventilations, then the tube is correctly inserted in the trachea and not in the esophagus. If the color stays purple, then the tube is not correctly inserted in the trachea or it is in the esophagus. A simple way to remember this is "YELLOW for YES" and "PURPLE for POOR." Note: When saturated with secretions, the carbon dioxide detector may not give appropriate color changes.

- *Laryngoscope handle and blades.* The laryngoscope is used by the advanced provider to elevate the tongue and sweep it out of the way, which allows for visualization of the glottic opening (opening into the trachea). The laryngoscope consists of a handle and blade. Blades come in a variety of sizes ranging from 0 to 4 and are either curved (Macintosh) (Figure 2-3) or straight (Miller, Flagg, and Wisconsin) (Figure 2-4). The handle holds the batteries for the bulb that is located in the blade. The handle also has a clip that allows for the attachment of the blade. A Miller blade is preferred for use with infants and toddlers because of the anatomy of the infant's oral cavity—longer epiglottis and more anterior glottic opening—thus allowing better visualization of the vocal cords.

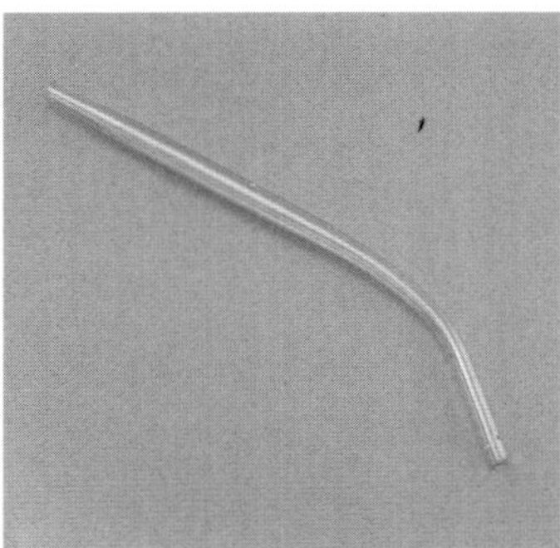

Figure 2-5 Rigid (tonsil-tip) suction catheter.

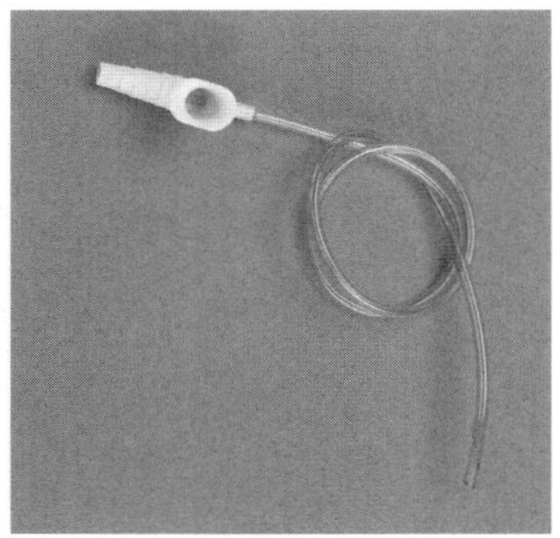

Figure 2-6 Whistle-tip suction catheter.

- *Oxygen.*
- *Pulse oximeter.*
- *Sharps container.*
- *Stethoscope.*
- *Stopwatch.*
- *Stylet.*
- *Tonsil-tip suction catheter.* A rigid tube used to clear secretions directly from the mouth and pharynx (Figure 2-5).
- *Water-soluble jelly.*
- *Whistle-tip suction catheter.* A narrow, flexible tube used to clear secretions through an ET tube or through the nasopharynx (Figure 2-6).

Preparation

- Examine all equipment, and test for defects.
- Ensure that the bulb for the laryngoscope is "light, bright, and tight." If it is not, change the battery in the handle. If the light is still not working, change handles or blades or both.

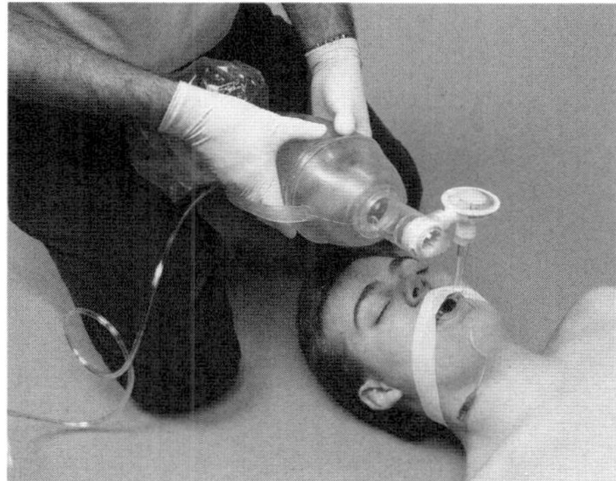

Figure 2-7 Orotracheal intubation.

- Check that the ET cuff will retain air by inflating the balloon with 10 mL of air. If the pilot balloon does not inflate, a rupture or a leak is present in the ET cuff. Change ET tube, and try again until the cuff is working properly. Be sure to deflate the cuff after checking.
- Lubricate the ET tube with water-soluble jelly.
- Wear appropriate personal protective equipment (PPE): goggles, face shield, gloves, and gown. Both the advanced and basic providers should wear appropriate PPE.

Procedure summary

Orotracheal intubation involves placing an ET tube through the mouth and into the trachea (Figure 2-7).

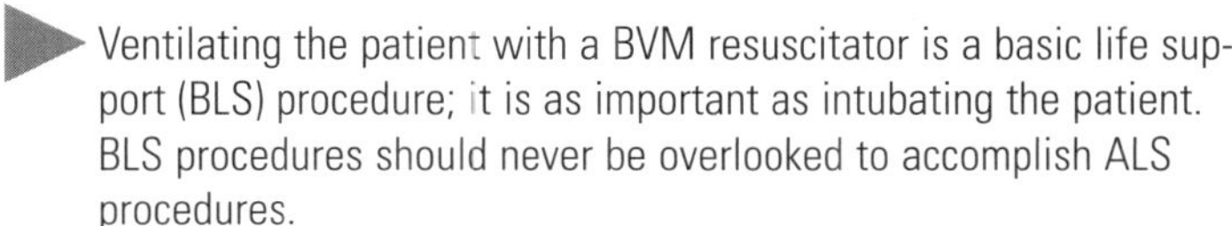

Ventilating the patient with a BVM resuscitator is a basic life support (BLS) procedure; it is as important as intubating the patient. BLS procedures should never be overlooked to accomplish ALS procedures.

Orotracheal Intubation

Orotracheal Intubation Steps

1. The nontrauma patient is placed in the sniffing position, and lungs are hyper-oxygenated with 100% oxygen for 1 to 2 minutes before intubation.

2. The advanced provider begins intubation.

BLS Provider Steps

1. Be prepared to ventilate by using a BVM resuscitator and to apply **cricoid pressure (Sellick's maneuver)** during BVM ventilation to avoid gastric distention. Note: The cricoid pressure should be discontinued only after appropriate insertion of the ET tube is confirmed. The companion CD-ROM to this text provides additional information on cricoid pressure.

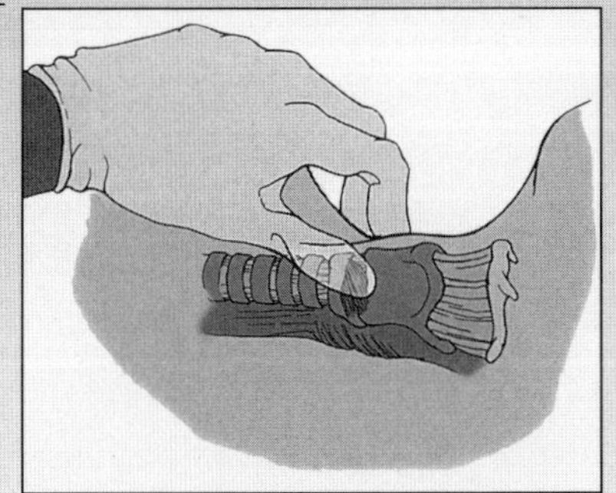

2. Prepare the following procedure.
   - Assemble suction unit with a tonsil-tip or whistle-tip suction catheter.

Orotracheal Intubation—cont'd

Orotracheal Intubation Steps	BLS Provider Steps
	• Attach laryngoscope blade to the handle. Ask which blade the advanced provider wishes to use; attach accordingly. • Place stylet into ET tube; if requested, form the tube into a J shape.
3. The advanced provider inserts the ET tube through the mouth into the trachea.	3. Prepare to perform the following: • Hand the ET tube to the advanced provider when asked. • Be a timer for the advanced provider. Let him or her know when 20 seconds approaches. • Apply cricoid pressure (Sellick's maneuver).
4. The patient is ventilated.	4. Prepare to resume ventilation with a bag-valve device (BVM unit without the mask): • Ensure that the mask has been removed from the BVM resuscitator after the patient is intubated. • Place the end-tidal CO_2 detector at the junction between the BVM resuscitator and ET tube. Note: The detector may be built into the BVM resuscitator.
5. The ET tube placement is confirmed.	5. Be prepared to perform the following: • Auscultate breath sounds over the **epigastrium** first. If the tube is in the appropriate place, no ventilation sounds should be

Continued

Orotracheal Intubation—cont'd

Orotracheal Intubation Steps	BLS Provider Steps
	heard. Listen bilaterally under the clavicles, under both nipples, and at the midaxillary line. Breath sounds should be heard equally over both lung fields. If breath sounds are heard only on the right side, the ET tube may have been inserted too far and may have entered the right mainstem bronchus. Alert the advanced provider of this finding. The advanced provider will deflate the cuff, pull back slightly on the tube, and then reinflate the cuff. Auscultate again to ensure that bilateral breath sounds are present. • Check for color change on the end-tidal CO_2 detector. Remember, "YELLOW for YES" and "PURPLE for POOR."
6. The airway is secured.	6. Be prepared to obtain or prepare the securing device or to maintain ventilation of the patient while the advanced provider secures the airway.
7. An ongoing assessment is necessary.	7. Be prepared to reaffirm tube placement at the request of the advanced provider. Note: ET tube placement should always be rechecked if the patient has been moved or if any change in the patient's condition has occurred.

On the Scene

You are on the scene dealing with a patient with apnea (not breathing). The advanced provider advises you to prepare for intubation while she works on stabilizing the patient. You will need an appropriately sized ET tube, stylet, laryngoscope blade and handle, 10 mL syringe, end-tidal carbon dioxide detector, and ET tube holder. While setting up the laryngoscope, you ask the advanced provider if she prefers the straight blade or curved blade and the size of blade that should be used. You also ensure the light on the blade is "light, bright, and tight." Finally, you check to ensure that there are no leaks in the cuff before handing the tube to the advanced provider. The advanced provider intubates the patient, and you assist by confirming breath sounds through auscultation.

NASOTRACHEAL INTUBATION

Nasotracheal intubation is an alternative method to orotracheal intubation (Figure 2-8). This method may be preferred over orotracheal intubation when the patient has clenched teeth or if motion of the cervical spine needs to be limited. The companion CD-ROM to this text provides additional information on nasotracheal intubation.

When will I see it?

- Patient needs aggressive airway management and is spontaneously breathing.
- Patient exhibits a gag reflex and is in respiratory distress (conscious or unconscious).
- Patient is experiencing trismus (clenched teeth).
- Patient has cervical spine injury.

When won't I see it?

- Patient has significant midface or head trauma.
- Patient is not spontaneously breathing.

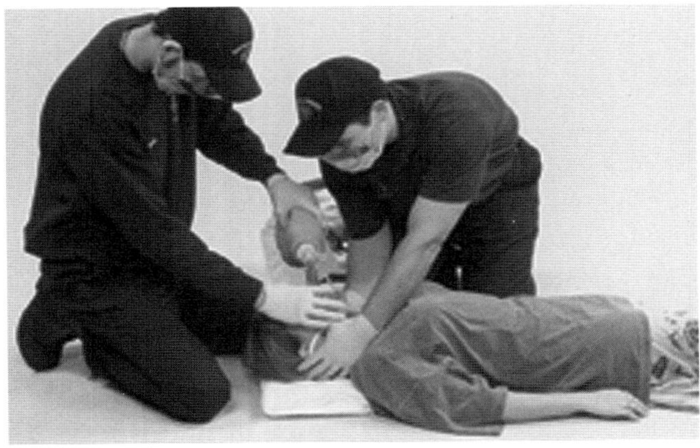

Figure 2-8 Nasotracheal intubation.

What should I watch for?

- Nose bleed
- Injury to the nasal septum
- Stimulation of the vagus nerve, thereby causing bradycardia
- Esophageal intubation
- Laceration of the pharynx upon insertion
- Timing; intubation attempt should only take 20 seconds

Equipment

- 10 mL syringe
- BVM resuscitator
- Cuffed ET tube, one size smaller than the tube that would be used for optimal orotracheal intubation
- ET tube holder
- End-tidal carbon dioxide detector
- Oxygen
- Sharps container
- Stethoscope
- Stopwatch
- Tonsil-tip suction catheter
- Water-soluble jelly
- Whistle-tip suction catheter

Preparation

- Examine all equipment, and test for defects.
- Check that the ET cuff will retain air by inflating the balloon with 10 mL of air. If the pilot balloon does not inflate, a rupture or a leak may be present in the ET cuff. Change the ET tube, and try again until the cuff is working properly. Be sure to deflate the cuff after checking and before handling it to the advanced provider.
- Lubricate the ET tube with water-soluble jelly.
- Wear appropriate PPE: goggles, face shield, gloves, and gown. Both the advanced and basic providers should wear appropriate PPE.

Nasotracheal Intubation

Nasotracheal Intubation Steps

1. The nontrauma patient is placed in the sniffing position, and lungs are hyper-oxygenated with 100% oxygen for 1 to 2 minutes before intubation.
2. The advanced provider begins intubation procedure.
3. The advanced provider inserts ET tube through the nose into the trachea.
4. The patient is ventilated.

BLS Provider Steps

1. Be prepared to ventilate by using a BVM resuscitator and to apply cricoid pressure (Seliick's maneuver) during BVM ventilation to avoid gastric distention. Note: The cricoid pressure should be discontinued only after appropriate insertion of the ET tube is confirmed.
2. Assemble the suction unit with a tonsil-tip or whistle-tip suction catheter.
3. Prepare the following:
   - Hand the ET tube to the advanced provider when asked.
   - Be a timer for the advanced provider. Let him or her know when 20 seconds is approaching.
   - Apply cricoid pressure (Sellick's maneuver).
4. Prepare to resume ventilation with a bag-valve device (BVM unit without the mask):
   - Ensure that the mask has been removed from the BVM resuscitator after the patient is intubated.
   - Place the end-tidal CO_2 detector at the junction between the BVM resuscitator and the ET tube. Note: The detector may be built into the BVM resuscitator.

Nasotracheal Intubation—cont'd

Nasotracheal Intubation Steps

5. The ET tube placement is confirmed.

6. The airway is secured.

7. An ongoing assessment is necessary.

BLS Provider Steps

5. Be prepared to perform the following:
   - Auscultate breath sounds over the epigastrium first. If the tube is in the appropriate place, no ventilation sounds will be heard. Listen bilaterally under the clavicles, under both nipples, and at the midaxillary line. Breath sounds should be equally heard over both lung fields. If breath sounds are heard only on the right side, the ET tube has probably been inserted too far and has entered the right mainstem bronchus. Alert the advanced provider of this finding. The advanced provider will deflate the cuff, pull back slightly on the tube, and reinflate the cuff. You should then auscultate again to ensure that bilateral breath sounds are present.
   - Check for color change on the end-tidal CO_2 detector. Remember, "YELLOW for YES" and "PURPLE for POOR."

6. Be prepared to obtain or prepare the securing device or to maintain ventilation while the advanced provider secures the patient's airway.

7. Be prepared to reaffirm tube placement at the request of the advanced provider. Note: ET tube placement should always be rechecked if the patient has been moved or if any change in the patient's condition has occurred.

On the Scene

You are assisting with a patient who is spontaneously breathing but is in severe respiratory distress. The advanced provider tells you to prepare for nasal intubation. You obtain the appropriately sized ET tube (smaller size than the tube used for orotracheal intubation), 10 mL syringe, end-tidal CO_2 detector, and ET tube holder. In addition, you apply water-soluble jelly to the tube before insertion. Finally, you check that there are no leaks in the cuff before handing the tube to the advanced provider. The advanced provider inserts the ET tube into one nostril and through the vocal cords into the trachea. After the advanced provider inserts the tube into the trachea, you assist by inflating the cuff, confirming breath sounds, or assuming ventilation responsibilities while the advanced provider assesses breath sounds and applies the end-tidal CO_2 detector.

ENDOTRACHEAL SUCTIONING

ET suctioning is the process of removing secretions, fluid, and other foreign objects from the lungs that are hampering ventilation and oxygenation (Figure 2-9). Preventing aspiration by inhalation is the main focus.

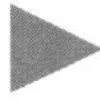

Remember, it is important for the patient to be well oxygenated before and after suctioning.

Advantage

* Suctions the tracheobronchial tree directly.

When will I see it?

* Respirations appear noisy (e.g., gurgling).
* Fluid is observed advancing up the ET tube.

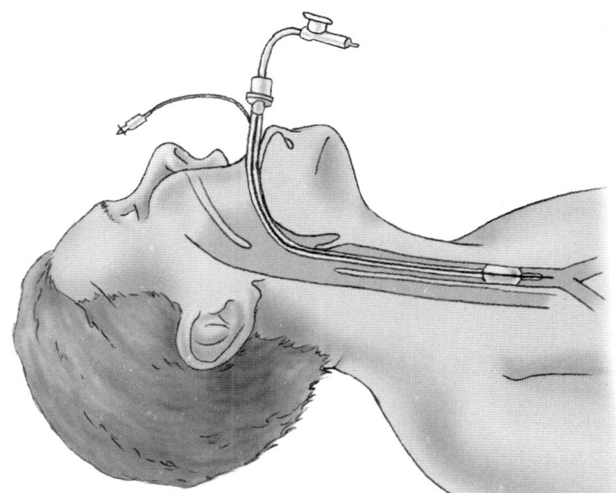

Figure 2-9 ET suctioning.

When won't I see it?

- Clear lung sounds are heard.
- Bradycardia is present.
- No tracheal, bronchial, or oropharyngeal secretions are present.

What should I watch for?

- Patient may become severely hypoxic, and dysrhythmias may result because of hypoxemia.
- Bradycardia as the result of stimulation of the vagus nerve.
- Suctioning should not exceed more than 10 to 15 seconds.

Equipment

- 10 mL syringe
- 3 to 5 mL of saline
- BVM resuscitator
- ET tube
- Pulse oximeter
- Oxygen
- Sharps container
- Stopwatch
- Suction device
- Tonsil-tip suction catheter
- Whistle-tip suction catheter

Preparation

- Examine all equipment, and test for defects.
- Turn on the suction device, and set it between -80 and -120 mm Hg.
- Wear appropriate PPE: goggles, face shield, gloves, and gown. Both the advanced and basic providers should wear appropriate PPE.

Procedure summary

The advanced provider will insert a suction device into the ET tube. Suction is applied while retracting the catheter in a rotating fashion. It is important that the patient be hyper-oxygenated both before and after suctioning because suctioning occurs as a result of negative pressure, which effectively "sucks" air out of the airway.

Endotracheal Suctioning

Endotracheal Suctioning Steps	BLS Provider Steps
1. The patient's lungs are hyper-oxygenated with 100% oxygen for 2 to 5 minutes.	1. Prepare to ventilate by using a BVM resuscitator.
2. The advanced provider begins suctioning procedure.	2. Be prepared to perform the following: • Attach suction unit to the appropriate catheter. • Fill a 10 mL syringe with saline in case thick secretions are present or at the request of the advanced provider.
3. The advanced provider inserts the catheter down the ET tube. Suction is intermittently applied, and the catheter is withdrawn in a rotating motion. To create suction, a finger is placed over the T-connector that is attached to the catheter.	3. Be prepared to perform the following: • Watch the pulse oximeter monitor (see Chapters 4 and 7) to ensure that the patient's condition remains stable. • Be a timer for the advanced provider. Suction should not exceed 10 to 15 seconds.
4. The patient is ventilated.	4. Prepare to resume ventilation using a BVM resuscitator.

On the Scene

You are assisting a patient who is in severe respiratory distress. The advanced provider successfully intubates the patient and requests orotracheal suction. You retrieve a suction catheter and attach it to the suction unit. The advanced provider applies the suction, and you assist by monitoring the suction time and the patient's heart rhythm. Remember, suction should not be applied longer than 10 to 15 seconds, and the patient's heart rhythm should be stable.

MAGILL FORCEPS

Magill forceps is a tool that may be used in the management of airway obstruction (Figure 2-10). The Magill forceps is an angulated scissors that can be used to grasp and remove an object from the trachea with direct visualization. Although the advanced provider will perform this procedure, the basic provider can assist by knowing where the Magill forceps are kept in the unit and anticipating when they may be used with an airway obstruction.

AIRWAY ALTERNATIVES

In addition to ET intubation, other alternatives to airway management are available. The basic provider may be asked to assist with a laryngeal mask airway, percutaneous transtracheal ventilation, or surgical airway. Only advanced providers should perform these skills; however, basic providers should check with their medical directors and local protocols regarding their involvement with these skills.

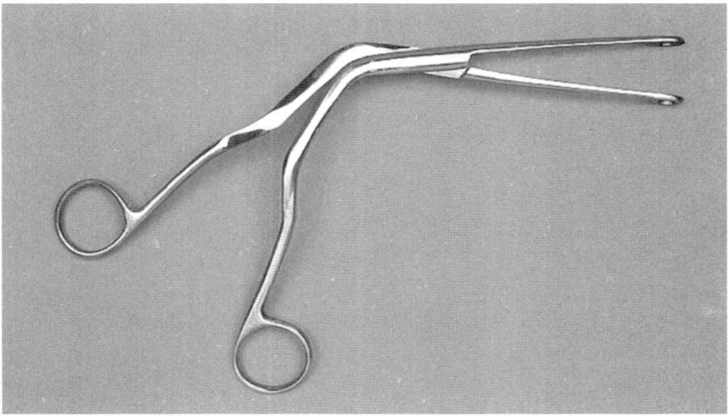

Figure 2-10 Magill forceps.

CHEST DECOMPRESSION

Chest (or pleural) decompression is the process used to expel air that is trapped in the pleural space as a result of chest or lung trauma or a ruptured bleb (a sac on the lung), which impedes cardiac and respiratory function (Figure 2-11). The companion CD-ROM to this text provides additional information on chest decompression.

When will I see it?

- Absent or decreased lung sounds are heard, along with signs and symptoms of a tension pneumothorax.

When won't I see it?

- Breath sounds are bilaterally present without signs of respiratory distress. No signs of a tension pneumothorax are observed.

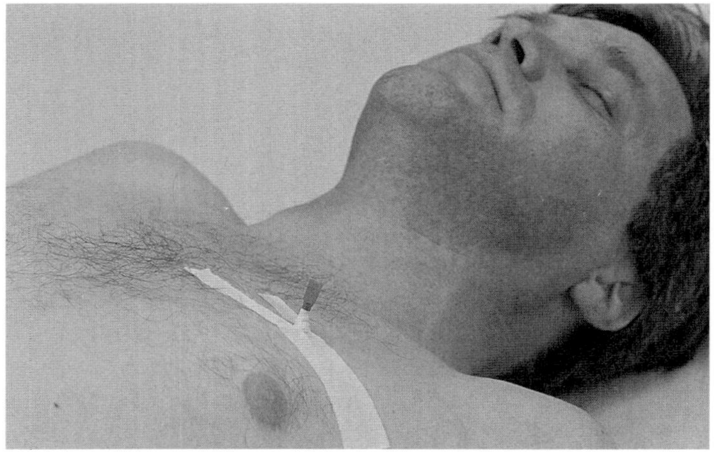

Figure 2-11 Chest decompression.

What should I watch for?

- Respiratory status improves after decompression.
- Mental status improves.
- Patient's color improves.
- Oxygenation improves.
- Blood pressure increases.
- Heart rate decreases.

Equipment

- 1 $^1/_2$ inch tape
- 14 or 16 gauge hollow IV needle
- 4 × 4 inch gauze pads
- Alcohol wipes or iodine
- BVM resuscitator
- Over-the-needle catheter
- Oxygen
- Sharps container
- Stethoscope

Preparation

- Wear appropriate PPE: goggles, face shield, gloves, and gown. Both the advanced and basic providers should wear appropriate PPE.

Procedure summary

The advanced provider inserts a needle into the affected side of the chest, allowing the trapped air to expel immediately.

Chest Decompression

Chest Decompression Steps	BLS Provider Steps
1. The advanced provider prepares the patient for procedure.	1. Retrieve a 14 or 16 gauge needle (size is determined by the advanced provider), an over-the-needle catheter, alcohol wipes, gauze, and tape.
2. The advanced provider auscultates the chest and evaluates the patient for signs and symptoms to reaffirm that a tension pneumothorax is present.	2. Prepare to ventilate using a BVM resuscitator and watch for the following: • Worsening respiratory distress • Increased resistance after ventilating • Systolic blood pressure <90 mm Hg • Decreased or absent breath sounds on one side during auscultation
3. The advanced provider inserts the needle into the chest on the affected side at the midclavicular line at the second or third intercostal space.	3. Prepare to perform the following: • Clean site with alcohol wipes or iodine. • Connect the needle to the catheter. • Listen for a rush of air as the needle is inserted into the chest, which indicates a release of pressure in the thorax surrounding the lung. • Auscultate for increased breath sounds after the insertion of the needle.
4. The advanced provider removes the needle but leaves the catheter in place and secures it.	4. Help tape the catheter in place.

On the Scene

You are assisting with the treatment of a multitrauma patient. The advanced provider assesses the patient and asks you to prepare for chest decompression. The patient is restless, has absent breath sounds on the right side of the chest, is hypotensive, tachycardic, and cyanotic; the pulse oximeter is showing 88% saturation. As the advanced provider finds the appropriate landmark, you assist by getting a 2 inch, 14 gauge IV needle, Betadine or alcohol wipes to prepare the site, and tape to secure the catheter after insertion. The advanced provider inserts the IV catheter into the chest cavity to expel the trapped air surrounding the lung. The catheter is left in place, but the needle is removed and disposed of appropriately.

Basic Electrocardiography

Objectives

After completing this chapter, you will be able to:
1. *Define the listed key terms.*
2. *Explain the basic electrical conduction system of the heart.*
3. *Identify and explain the different components to the electrocardiographic monitor.*
4. *Demonstrate electrode placement.*
5. *Identify the common electrocardiographic rhythms.*

Key Terms

Bundle branches *Branches of specialized electrical conducting cells that extend from the bundle of His into the ventricles, dividing into three branches.*

Bundle of His *Cardiac fibers that connect the atrioventricular node and the two bundle branches.*

Defibrillation *The discharge of electricity from a medical device into the chest when the heart has unstable or dysfunctional electrical activity.*

Diaphoresis *Excessive sweating.*

External cardiac pacing *Electrical pacing with a medical device that replaces or overrides existing dysfunctional cardiac electrical activity.*

Foci *Specific locations; that is, locations where electrical activity occur in the heart.*

Lead *Electrical connection attached to the body for the purpose of monitoring physiologic electrical activity.*

Myocardium *Thick middle layer of the heart.*

P wave *Represents atrial depolarization.*

PR interval *Represents the length of time required for the atria to depolarize and the delay of the impulse through the atrioventricular junction. Normally, the PR interval measures 0.12 to 0.20 seconds.*

QRS complex *Represents ventricular depolarization.*
- *Q wave is the first negative, downward, deflection after the P wave.*
- *R wave is the first positive, upward after the P wave.*
- *S wave is the negative deflection after the R wave.*
- *QRS complex usually measures 0.04 to 0.12 seconds.*

Synchronized cardioversion *Discharge of electricity from a medical device into the chest. It is synchronized with ventricular depolarization to convert an unstable rapid cardiac rhythm to a stable normal (sinus) heart rhythm.*

T wave *Represents ventricular repolarization.*

Transcutaneous cardiac pacing *See External cardiac pacing.*

INTRODUCTION

This section does not replace a formal ECG interpretation course. It may, however, serve as a starting point. The goal is to allow the basic provider to become familiar with common ECG rhythms and focus on the more lethal rhythms.

To understand ECG interpretation, it is important to become familiar with the electrical flow of the heart. As you may recall from Chapter 1, the SA node serves as the main pacemaker in the heart and is located in the right atrium.

Once the electrical impulse is discharged from the SA node, it travels through a variety of pathways throughout the atria until it reaches the AV junction (middle part of the heart). The impulse then travels through the AV node downward through the bundle of His and into the left and right bundle branches, two separate pathways of specialized cells that will allow the impulse to reach both ventricles independently of each other. Finally, the Purkinje fibers are similar specialized cells that project from the bundle branches into the myocardium and stimulate the mechanical cells, which promote myocardial contraction. This electrical activity is observed on the ECG monitor and only represents the electrical activity of the heart. It does not tell how well the heart is contracting. If you look at a normal ECG waveform (Figure 3-1), you will be able to pick out certain waves that represent some of the sites just

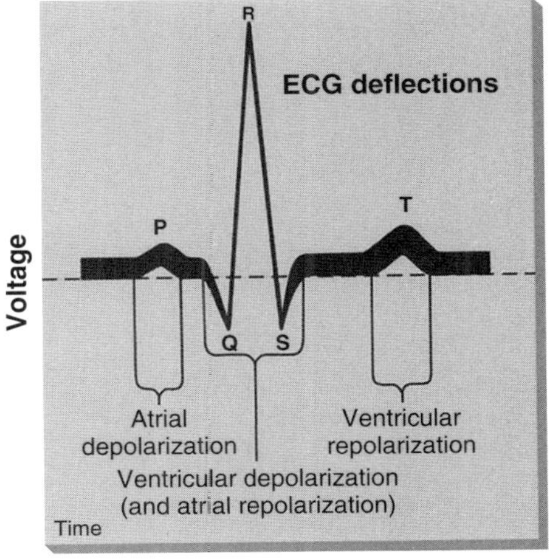

Figure 3-1 ECG waveform.

discussed, as well as in Chapter 1. To learn more about ECG interpretation refer to the "Suggested Readings" section at the back of this book.

ADVANCED LIFE SUPPORT FOR BASIC LIFE SUPPORT PROCEDURES

ECG APPLICATION

The ECG monitor is a vital component of the ALS Passport. The monitor provides the information needed to address a variety of cardiac issues: irregular heart rhythms, bradycardic and tachycardic rhythms, lethal rhythms such as ventricular fibrillation, and ischemic changes (changes noted on the ECG that indicate a lack of oxygen to the myocardium). The ECG monitor is not only used for ECG interpretation, but it is also used for defibrillation, synchronized cardioversion, and transcutaneous pacing. You can assist by becoming familiar with the ECG monitor used in your area. The ECG monitor is a vital tool for cardiac ALS and should be applied to all unstable or potentially unstable patients, especially when an irregular, slow, fast, or absent pulse is felt, if chest pain or shortness of breath is present, if the patient is unconscious or unresponsive, or if pallor or diaphoresis is present. The companion CD-ROM to this text provides additional information on cardiac monitoring and defibrillation.

Remember that the ALS Passport generally consists of the five essential components that need to be carried out on all unstable or potentially unstable patients before or during transport to the hospital: (1) oxygen administration, (2) IV line, (3) pulse oximetry, (4) ECG application, and (5) glucose check (depending on your local protocols).

When will I see it?

- Patients who are experiencing any of the following:
  - ▸ Chest pressure
  - ▸ Syncope (fainting)
  - ▸ Diaphoresis (excessive sweating)
  - ▸ Dyspnea (difficulty breathing)
  - ▸ Fast, slow, or no heart rate
  - ▸ Unstable blood pressure
  - ▸ Dizziness
  - ▸ Any sign or symptoms indicating that the patient is unstable or potentially unstable
- Defibrillation (ventricular fibrillation)
- Transcutaneous pacing (bradycardia $<$ 60 bpm with signs or symptoms of hypoperfusion)
- Synchronized cardioversion (tachycardia $>$160 bpm)
- Patients with a history of diabetes

When won't I see it?

- The ECG monitor may be applied on any patient.

What should I watch for?

- Irregular heart beat.
- Tachycardia (heart rate $>$ 100 beats/min).
- Bradycardia (heart rate $<$ 60 beats/min).
- Poor electrical activity on the monitor. Patient movement, muscle tremors, or electrical interference from an electrical source, such as a refrigerator, halogen lamps, and ceiling fans in close proximity of the monitor, may cause poor electrical activity.
- Loose cable.

Equipment

- *Alcohol wipes.*
- *Cardiac monitor.* The cardiac monitor consists of a screen, two defibrillation paddles or pads, and cables. In addition,

some monitors have a pacer function. Some monitors also have detachable paddles with a rotary dial on one of the paddles, which indicates 5 to 360 joules of electricity. Other monitors do not have paddles; they have what is referred to as *hands-off defibrillation.* These monitors have a cable that attaches to a set of pads that are used to defibrillate. Some pads are multifunctional and allow the advanced provider to defibrillate, synchronize cardiovert, and externally pace a patient with the same pads.

The cardiac monitor is also used for monitoring the electrical activity of the heart by applying color-coded cables onto sticky electrodes that are placed on the patient's skin. Most commonly, three electrodes are applied to the patient's body. One electrode is placed on the upper right chest, the second is placed on the upper left chest, and the third is applied on the left lower chest. An alternative placement is one electrode on the right arm, one on the left arm, and one on the left leg (Figure 3-2). The following buttons can be found on the monitor:

a. **Code summary.** When pressed, this button will print all cardiac events that were marked throughout the patient's care. (To mark a strip, press the record button on and then off when a rhythm is displayed.)

b. **ECG size.** Adjusts the size of the complexes.

c. **ECG volume.** Adjusts the volume. A tone is projected with every QRS complex.

d. **Record.** Records the rhythm displayed on the monitor. When pressed, this button will mark the specific event, which can later be retrieved through the code summary function. Some monitors have only a print button instead of a record button.

e. **Sync.** When pressed, this button allows the patient to be shocked at intervals synchronized with the patient's existing heart rhythm.

f. **Lead.** Allows for different leads or different views of the heart to be shown.

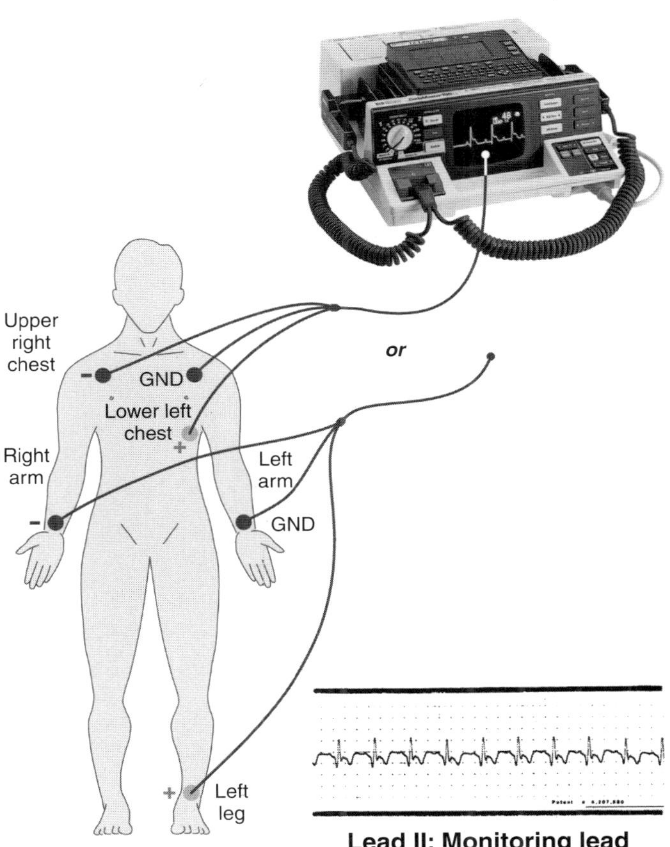

Figure 3-2 Electrode placement.

g. **Battery indicator.** Consists of three lights that are on when the unit is on. If a battery is low, a light will indicate which battery is low and a tone will be projected.

h. **Freeze button.** When pressed, this button is used to hold the rhythm being displayed in place for analysis.

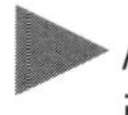 All monitors are different, and familiarization is key to understanding their functions.

Preparation

- Examine all equipment, and check for defects.
- Wear appropriate PPE: goggles, face shield, gloves, and gown. Both the advanced and basic providers should wear appropriate PPE.

Procedure summary

Many features are offered on the cardiac monitor; however, familiarity with your department's monitor will help prevent any delay in care. The monitor may be reviewed every morning during equipment "check out." In addition, an advanced provider can review the monitor features with you.

ECG Application

ECG Application Steps	BLS Provider Steps
1. Prepare the patient for electrode application.	1. For electrode placement, prepare to cleanse the skin with alcohol to remove body oil and dirt.
2. Place the electrodes to the patient's skin and attaches the cables to the electrodes.	2. Be prepared to place the electrodes on the right and left upper chest and left lower chest or other placement, depending on the preference of the advanced provider. Note: Most commonly, the white colored cable goes to the right shoulder, the black cable goes to the left shoulder, and the red cable is attached to the lower extremity.

ECG Application—cont'd

ECG Application Steps	BLS Provider Steps
3. The ECG monitor is turned on, appropriate view is selected, and baseline heart rhythm is obtained.	3. Turn on the monitor, and select the appropriate view. Note: Generally, lead II is used unless another view is requested. If the signal is poor, recheck the cable connections and electrode placement on the patient's skin. A poor signal can be caused by excessive body hair, perspiration, dried conductive gel, and poor electrode placement.

EXTERNAL CARDIAC PACING

External cardiac pacing, also known as transcutaneous cardiac pacing, is an effective emergency therapy for asystole, complete heart block, bradycardia, and suppression of some life-threatening rhythms. This emergency therapy involves the delivery of electrical currents to the heart by using a pacemaking device. The device substitutes for the natural pacemaker within the heart that has become dysfunctional or blocked.

When will I see it?

- Patient with bradycardia, resulting in hypotension (may be helpful during early asystolic arrest)
- Patient with second- or third-degree heart block, resulting in hypoperfusion

When won't I see it?

- Rhythms other than bradycardia
- Bradycardia with no signs of hypoperfusion

What should I watch for?

- Increase in blood pressure

Equipment

- Alcohol wipes
- ECG monitor and cables
- Pacing pads

Preparation

- Examine all equipment, and check for defects.
- Wear appropriate PPE: goggles, face shield, gloves, and gown. Both the advanced and basic providers should wear appropriate PPE.

Procedure summary

The advanced provider determines when to initiate external pacing and sets the amount of energy to be delivered to the patient. Many monitors can provide external pacing. Once pacing is determined, two pads are applied to the patient's torso in an anteroposterior or anteroanterior position (Figure 3-3). The pads provide a conductive medium that allows the delivery of electrical energy to the heart. The transcutaneous

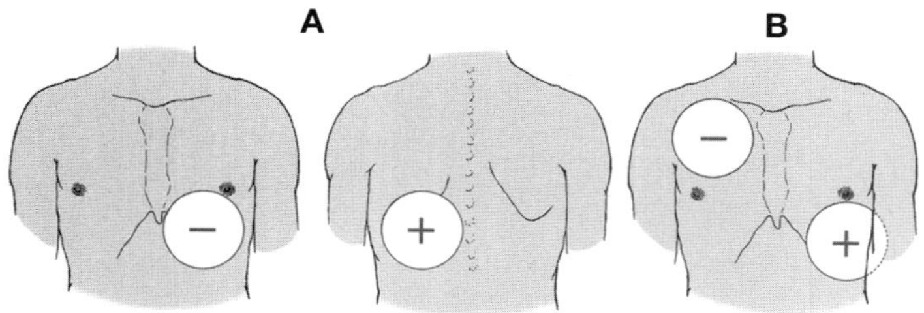

Figure 3-3 **A,** Anteroposterior positioning of transcutaneous electrode pads. **B,** Anterolateral positioning of transcutaneous electrode pads.

pacer is used for patients who have low blood pressure with signs and symptoms of hypoperfusion (shock) as a result of a slow heart rate (bradycardia <60 bpm). When applied, the transcutaneous pacer may increase the patient's heart rate, thereby elevating the patient's blood pressure.

External Cardiac Pacing

External Cardiac Pacing Steps	BLS Provider Steps
1. The advanced provider explains the procedure to the patient. He or she connects the patient to the monitor, obtains a rhythm strip, and determines baseline vital signs.	1. Set up the monitor, and cleanse the area of skin for electrode placement with alcohol to remove body oil and dirt.
2. The advanced provider applies electrodes to the patient and attaches the pacing cables and pacing device.	2. Be prepared to place the two pacing electrodes in proper position, turn on the pacer, and ensure it is set to pacing. *Anteroposterior:* • Place the negative pad and negative pacer wire on the left anterior chest, halfway between the xiphoid process and left nipple, with the upper edge of the electrode below the nipple line. • Place the positive pad and positive pacer wire on the left posterior chest beneath the scapula lateral to the spine on the left side.

External Cardiac Pacing—cont'd

External Cardiac Pacing Steps	BLS Provider Steps
	Anteroanterior: • Place the negative pad between the right nipple and clavicle. • Place the positive pad over the anterolateral region just below the left nipple. Pacing mode is also determined.
3. The advanced provider selects the pacing rate and current.	3. Set the rate (usually 70 bpm) to the number indicated by the advanced provider, and set the current (begin with 50 milliamps).
4. The pacemaker is activated, and the patient and ECG are observed. Rhythm strips are obtained as appropriate. The advanced provider anticipates further therapy.	4. Monitor ECG and the patient for vital signs.

On the Scene

You are on the scene assisting with a patient who is apneic and pulseless. BLS is immediately initiated, and the advanced provider asks you to apply the ECG monitor. Because this patient is pulseless, the application of the multipurpose pads is indicated for immediate defibrillation. You have applied the pads, one between the right clavicle and right nipple and one under the left nipple (anterolateral) to obtain a quick look. This quick look allows you to rapidly ascertain the patient's cardiac rhythm. The monitor displays the rhythm shown below.

You recognize the rhythm as ventricular fibrillation, and immediate electrical defibrillation is needed. The advanced provider sets the energy setting to 200 joules and defibrillates immediately. Once the defibrillation is complete, you assist with securing an airway, providing IV access, and preparing medications.

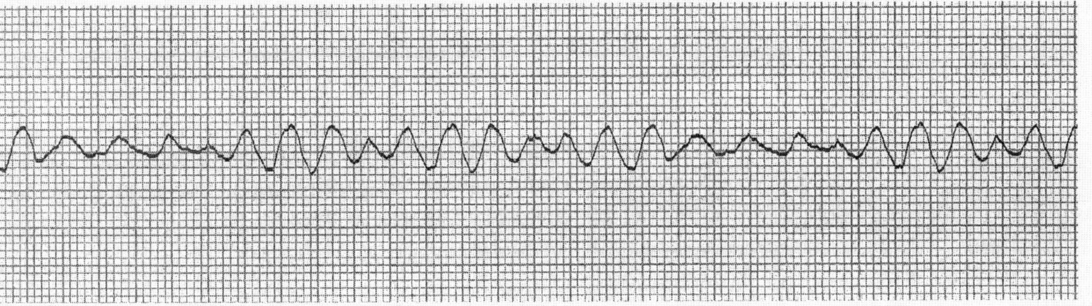

On the Scene

You are assisting with a 56-year-old woman who is complaining of dizziness. The patient's vital signs are blood pressure 72/56, heart rate 44, and respiratory rate 24. The patient's skin is cool and pale. The ECG monitor reveals the rhythm shown below. The advanced provider alerts you that the patient is bradycardic and has signs and symptoms of hypo-perfusion. In addition, the advanced provider requests the application of the transcutaneous pacer. You assist by placing the negative pad and negative pacer wire on the left anterior chest, halfway between the xiphoid process and left nipple, with the upper edge of the electrode below the nipple line. You place the positive pad and positive pacer wire on the left posterior chest beneath the scapula and lateral to the spine. You turn the pacer on and set the rate at 70 bpm as requested by the advanced provider. The advanced provider sets the amount of energy to be delivered to the patient. Once the patient is paced, you assist by assessing vital signs and working with the advanced provider to secure an airway and IV access and to prepare medication.

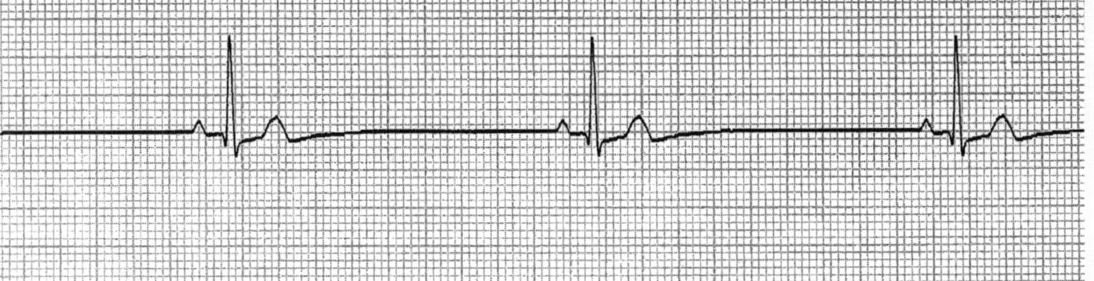

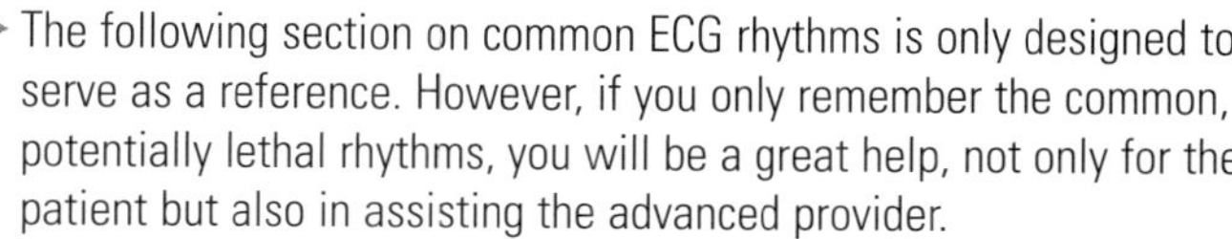

The following section on common ECG rhythms is only designed to serve as a reference. However, if you only remember the common, potentially lethal rhythms, you will be a great help, not only for the patient but also in assisting the advanced provider.

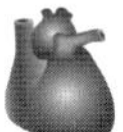

Note: These potentially lethal rhythms will be marked with a heart icon.

In general, look out for fast rates, slow rates, or no rate at all. You don't have to memorize all the ECG rhythms, but if you can detect a slow heart rate (<60 bpm) or a fast heart rate (>100 bpm) by taking a pulse, it will be a great help. Remember that tachycardia equals fast (>100 bpm) and bradycardia equals slow (<60 bpm). Importantly, rates will vary in the pediatric age group. For example, a heart rate of 100 bpm may be normal for an infant or a child.

COMMON ECG RHYTHMS

Normal sinus rhythm

Everything looks good here. The SA node is the pacemaker and is firing at a regular rate of 60 to 100 bpm. Every impulse is being conducted from the atria to the ventricles. This is what a normal ECG should look like (Figure 3-4).

Regularity. R-R intervals are constant, and the rhythm is regular.

Rate. Atrial and ventricular rates are equal and between 60 and 100 bpm.

P wave. A noticeable P wave can be seen before every complex and within the normal PR interval.

PRI. PR interval is between 0.12 and 0.20 seconds.

QRS complex. QRS complex measures less than 0.12 seconds.

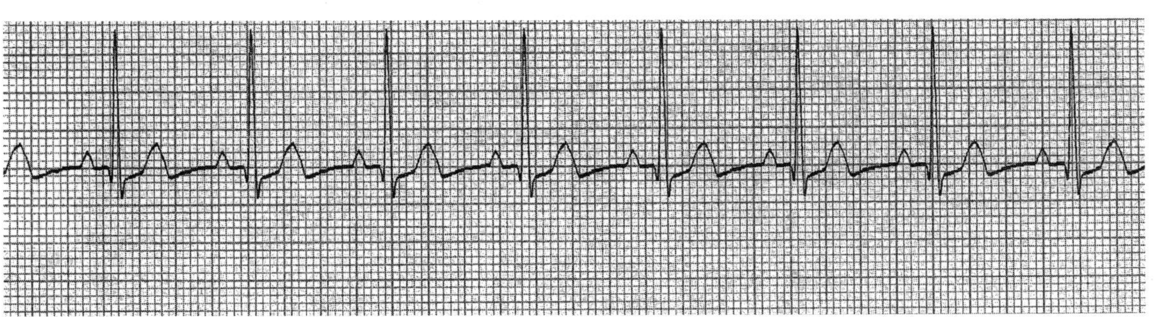

Figure 3-4 Normal sinus rhythm.

Sinus bradycardia

The rate is a little too slow for my taste. The SA node is the pacemaker, but it is firing at a rate less than 60 bpm (Figure 3-5). Signs and symptoms are the key factors when determining whether a slow heart rate is too slow. It is not uncommon for individuals who are athletes to have a resting heart rate less than 60 bpm. Nevertheless, if a patient has a heart rate less than 60 bpm and is hypotensive or is experiencing chest pain, shortness of breath, diaphoresis, or dizziness, the patient is considered unstable.

Regularity. R-R interval is normal, and the rhythm is regular.

Rate. Rate is less than 60 bpm.

P wave. Uniform P wave can be seen before every QRS complex.

PRI. PR interval is normal, 0.12 to 0.20 seconds.

QRS. QRS complex is less than 0.12 seconds.

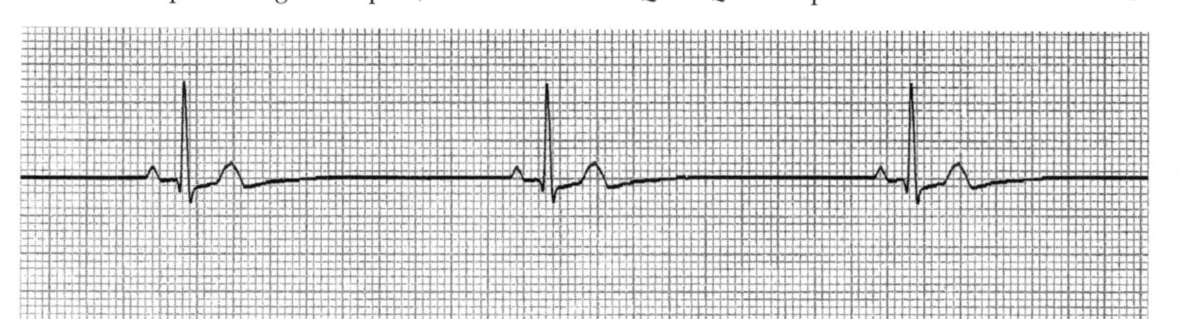

Figure 3-5 Sinus bradycardia.

Sinus tachycardia

Buckle up, we're going for a ride. The SA node is the pacemaker. It is firing at a rate greater than 100 bpm (Figure 3-6).

Sinus tachycardia may represent a variety of underlying problems. Count the number of R waves in 6 seconds, and multiply that number by 10. If it is over 100, it is a tachycardic rhythm.

Regularity. Rhythm is normal.

Rate. Rate is greater than 100 bpm and can be between 100 and 160 bpm.

P wave. P wave is present and in front of every QRS complex.

PRI. PR interval is between 0.12 and 0.20 seconds.

QRS. QRS complex is less than 0.12 seconds.

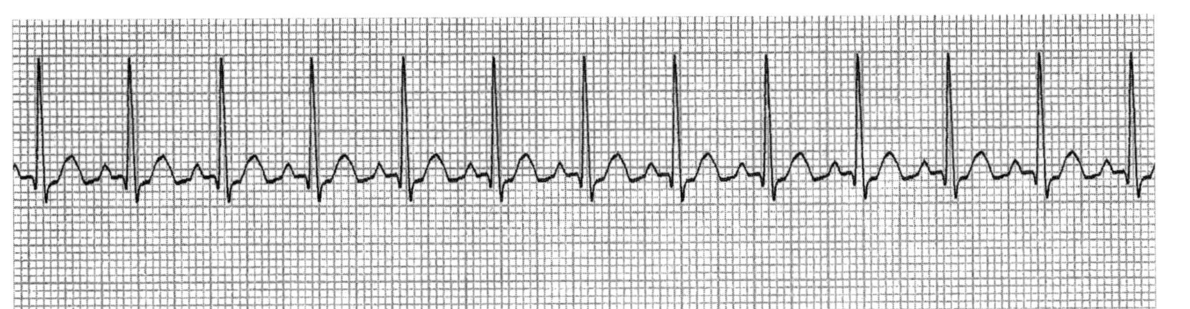

Figure 3-6 Sinus tachycardia.

Premature atrial contractions

Don't jump ahead, wait your turn. The premature beat is generated by an irritable focus within the atria, which fires prematurely and causes an abnormal beat (Figure 3-7). Conduction through the ventricles is normal. In this situation, an irritable site in the atria decides to fire before the SA node, thereby causing an irregular beat.

Regularity. Rhythm is slightly irregular because of premature beats.

Rate. Rate may vary.

P wave. P wave may be present, but it will have a different morphology.

PRI. PR intervals may vary because of the extra focus in the atria.

QRS. Measurement is within normal limits.

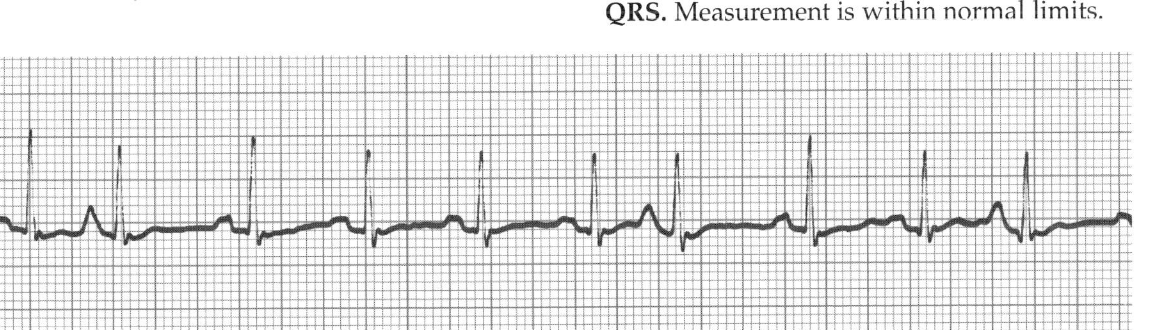

Figure 3-7 Sinus tachycardia with three premature atrial contractions (PACs). From left to right, beats 2, 7, and 10 are PACs.

Atrial tachycardia

Hey, what happen to Mr. SA node? An irritable focus in the atria is firing at a very rapid rate (Figure 3-8). Conduction through the ventricles is normal. If you look closely, the P waves, if visible, will not appear as rounded as you see when the impulse originates from the SA node. The rate is tachycardic and originates in the atria.

Regularity. Rhythm may be slightly irregular because the origin of the impulse is different from the main pacemaker; irritable foci.

Rate. Rate may be anywhere between 150 and 250 bpm.

P wave. P wave is seen in front of every QRS, but it may be hidden in the preceding T wave because of the rapid rate. The morphology will be different.

PRI. PR interval is constant, 0.12 to 0.20 seconds. It will be very difficult to distinguish because of the rapid rate.

QRS. QRS complex is less than 0.12 seconds.

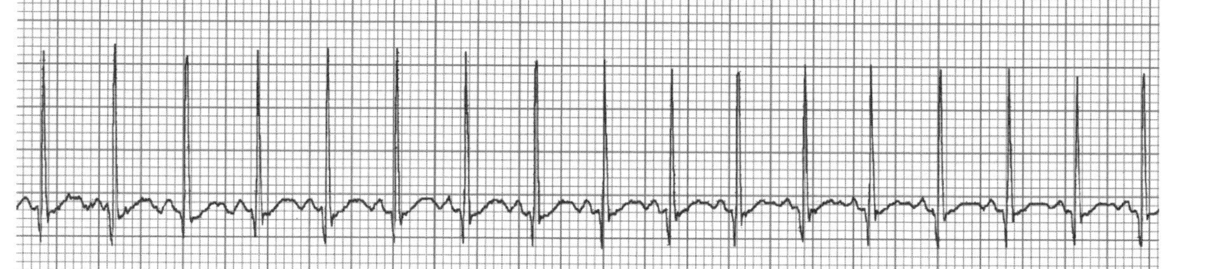

Figure 3-8 Atrial tachycardia.

Atrial flutter

Do you like my look? It is called the saw-tooth look. Irritable foci in the atria are firing at very rapid rates. A blocking mechanism at the AV node is reducing the amount of impulses being sent into the ventricles (Figure 3-9).

Regularity. Atrial rhythm is regular, but the ventricular rhythm may be irregular, depending on the type of conduction pattern.

Rate. Atrial rate is between 250 and 350 bpm. Ventricular rate depends on the type of conduction.

P wave. Atrial flutter will create noticeable P waves. When examined closely, they have a saw-tooth appearance.

PRI. PR interval is not measured in atrial flutter because of the close proximity to the QRS.

QRS. Measures 0.12 seconds if no P waves are concealed in the QRS wave.

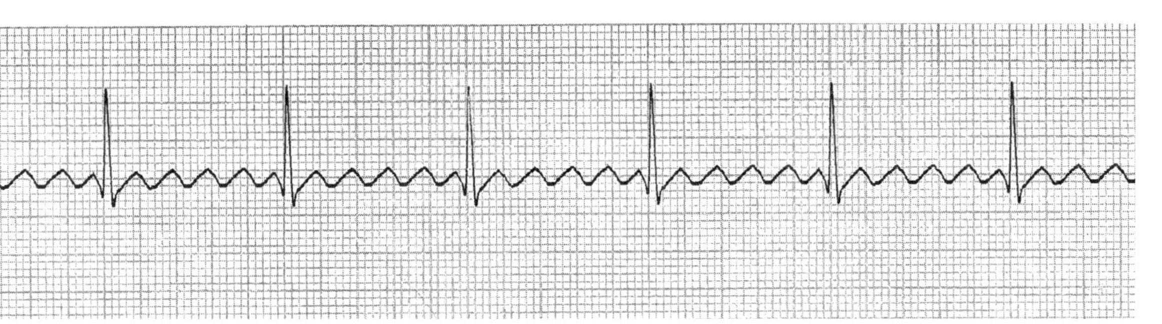

Figure 3-9 Atrial flutter.

Atrial fibrillation

Why are the atria so upset? I liked it better when the SA node was in charge and the ventricular beats were all regular. A variety of irritable foci are in the atria. Therefore the atria are continuously depolarized. A blocking mechanism at the AV node level helps the ventricles receive impulses at an acceptable rate (Figure 3-10).

Regularity. Atria are firing at such a fast rate that they are fibrillating. The ventricles are depolarized in an irregular pattern.

Rate. Atrial rate may exceed 350 bpm. The ventricular rate is usually below 100 bpm. If the rate is higher than 100 bpm, it is a rapid ventricular response.

P wave. P waves are displayed as fibrillatory waves with no measurable pattern.

PRI. No P waves are visible; no PR interval can be measured.

QRS. QRS complex is less than 0.12 seconds.

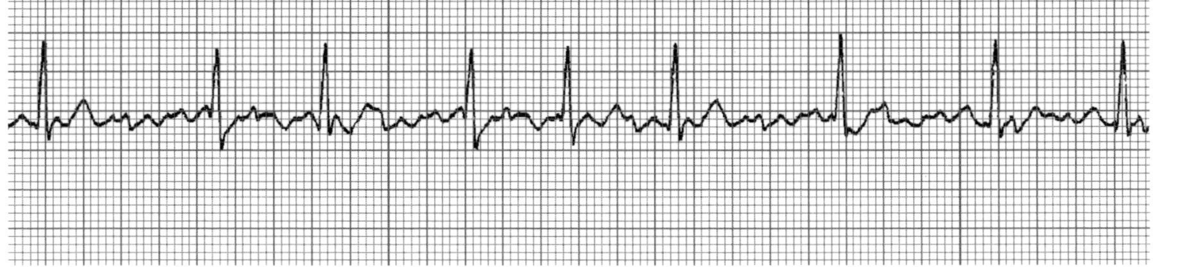

Figure 3-10 Atrial fibrillation.

Junctional escape rhythm

I hate it when the SA node falls asleep, now I have to work. When the main pacemaker fails, the AV node will assume the responsibility of producing an impulse (Figure 3-11). During this phase, the impulse will not only travel toward the ventricles, but it will also travel toward the atria in a retrograde fashion.

Regularity. Rhythm is regular.

Rate. Rate is usually between 40 and 60 bpm.

P waves. No evidence of a P wave is observed in the QRS. P wave may be seen in front of the QRS, but it is inverted. It may be found after the QRS.

PRI. No PR intervals may be observed. If the P wave appears before the QRS, it will be less than 0.12 seconds.

QRS. QRS complex is less than 0.12 seconds.

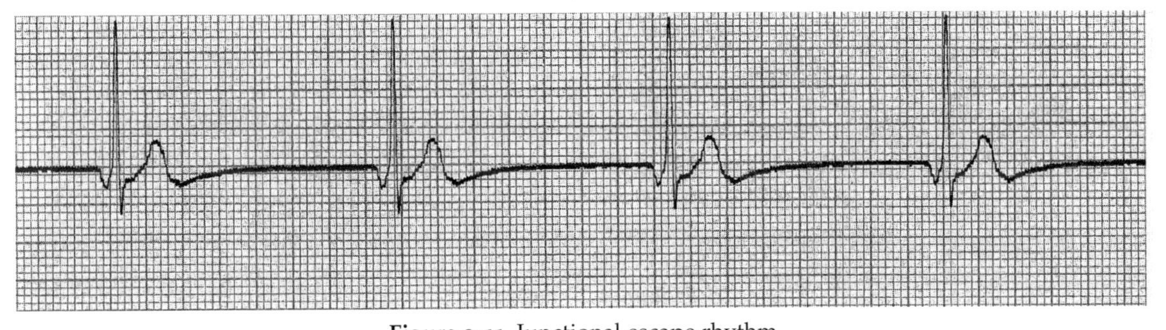

Figure 3-11 Junctional escape rhythm.

Accelerated junctional rhythm

Who says I can't initiate impulses as fast as the SA node? An irritable focus in the AV junction overrides the SA node and creates a retrograde conduction into the atria. Conduction into the ventricles is normal (Figure 3-12).

Regularity. Rhythm is regular.

Rate. Rate is between 60 and 100 bpm.

P waves. P waves are inverted and can come before, during, or after the QRS complex.

PRI. PR interval is less than 0.12 seconds when it falls before the QRS.

QRS. QRS complex is less than 0.12 seconds.

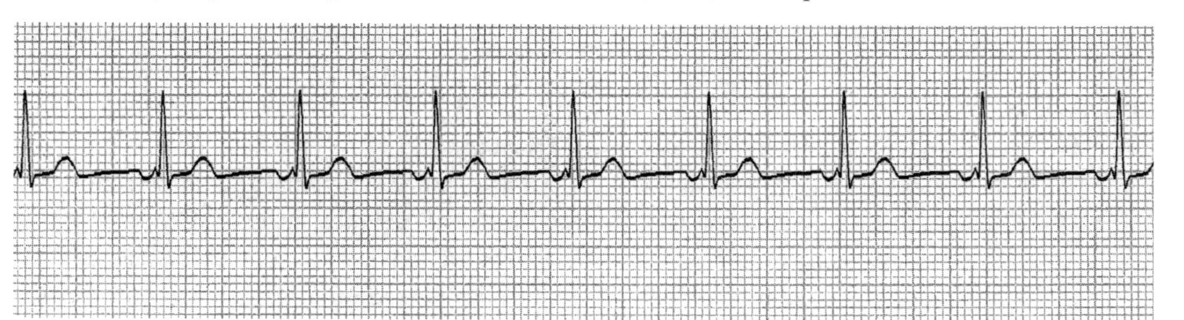

Figure 3-12 Accelerated junctional rhythm.

Junctional tachycardia

Don't get me confused with sinus tachycardia. He has an upright P wave, and I don't. An irritable focus in the AV junction overrides the SA node. The impulse is initiated retrograde into the atria, but it is conducted into the ventricles via the normal route (Figure 3-13).

Regularity. Rhythm is regular, and R-R are constant.

Rate. Rate will be over 100 bpm; atrial and ventricular rates are the same.

P waves. P waves can come before, during, or after the QRS waves and are inverted with PR intervals less than 0.12 seconds.

PRI. PR interval is less than 0.12 seconds.

QRS. QRS complex measures less than 0.12 seconds.

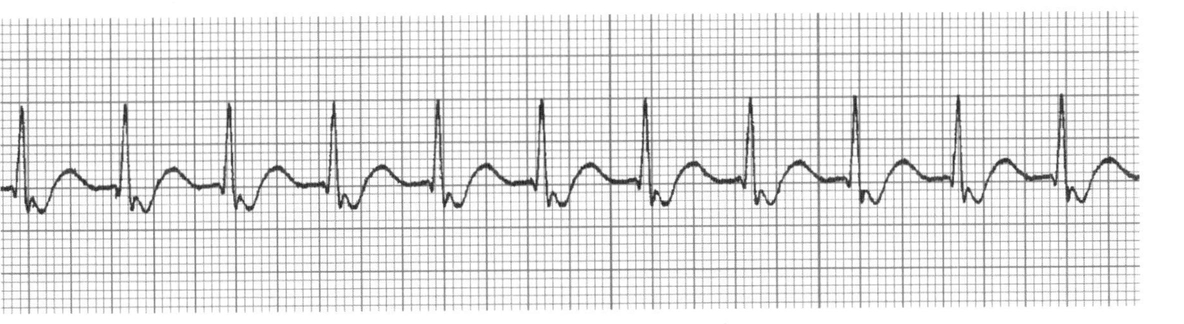

Figure 3-13 Junctional tachycardia.

First-degree heart block

Will you stop talking with the AV gate keeper and deliver the message to the ventricles? The impulse is initiated by the SA node and travels through the AV node. It is detained there for sometimes longer than 0.20 seconds. Once it clears the AV node, the impulse travels through the ventricles as normal (Figure 3-14). Imagine driving up to a toll booth and placing your money in the basket. It takes awhile for the arm to lift; you are detained for a couple of seconds. Once the arm goes up, you go on your way without any problems.

Regularity. Rate is regular but depends on the delay.

Rate. Rate is usually between 60 and 100 bpm.

P wave. P wave is present and upright.

PRI. PR interval is delayed longer than 0.20 seconds.

QRS. QRS is less than 0.12 seconds.

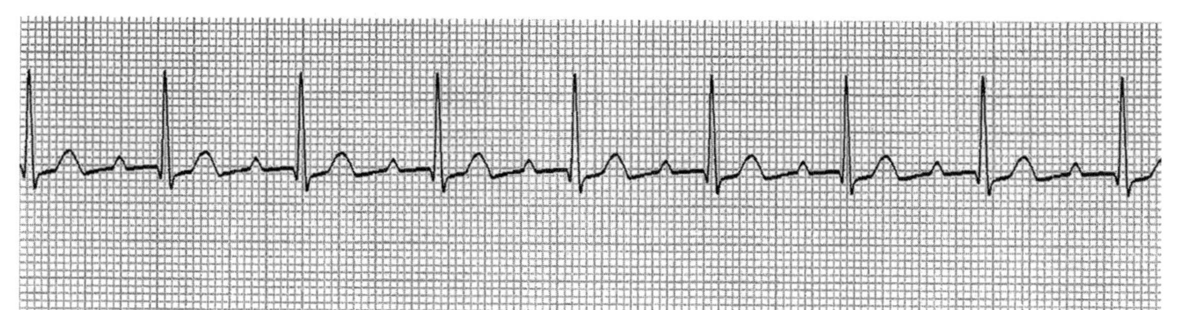

Figure 3-14 First-degree heart block.

Second-degree heart block, type 1 (Wenckebach)

Going, going, gone.... The atria initiate an impulse. It is delayed once it reaches the AV node but then is sent on its way (Figure 3-15). Assessing the PRI as it gets progressively longer and as the QRS wave is eventually dropped is the key. Three or more consecutive complexes are needed to determine a Wenckebach. This rhythm tricks many practitioners. Always check the PR interval, which will reveal information, especially when dealing with heart blocks. The PR interval will lengthen until a QRS complex is dropped.

Regularity. Rhythm is regularly irregular.

Rate. Rate is usually between 60 and 100 bpm.

P waves. P waves are present and upright. Some may not be followed by a QRS.

PRI. PR intervals get progressively longer, until the QRS wave is dropped.

QRS. QRS complex is less than 0.12 seconds and is occasionally dropped.

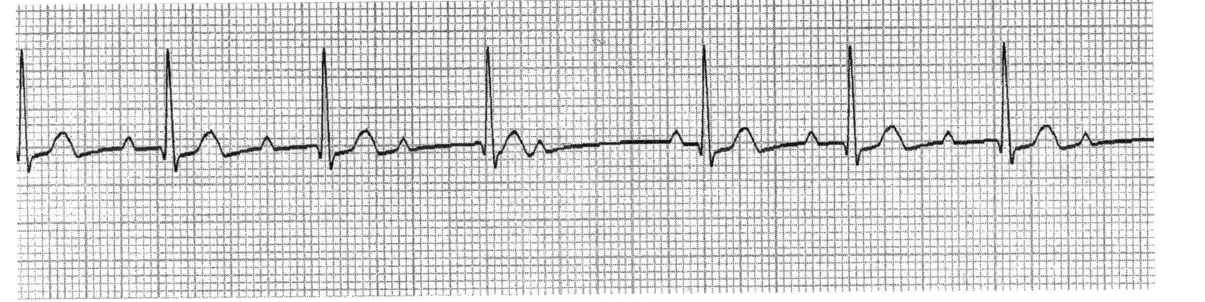

Figure 3-15 Second-degree heart block, type 1.

Second-degree heart block, type 2

Hey, why so many P waves? The atria send an impulse, but it is detained at the AV node. Therefore another impulse is sent and travels through the AV node without any problems into the ventricles (Figure 3-16). The key is to look at the PR intervals. The P wave that precedes the QRS wave has a regular PR interval. One P wave will successfully make it through the AV junction, reaching the ventricles with a normal PR interval.

Regularity. Rhythm is regular.

Rate. Rate is usually between 60 and 100 bpm.

P wave. P wave is present and upright. More than one P wave is sent for every QRS complex.

PRI. PR interval is normal, 0.12 to 0.20 seconds. P wave precedes the QRS complex.

QRS. QRS complex is less than 0.12 seconds.

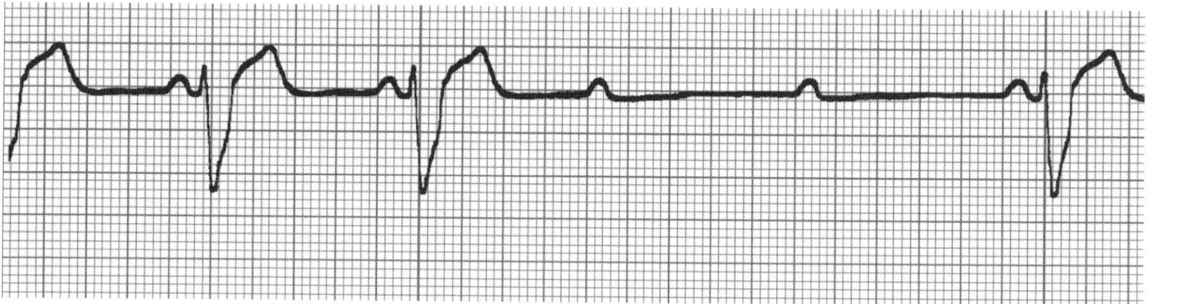

Figure 3-16 Second-degree heart block, type 2.

Third-degree (complete) heart block

What a mess. The atria and ventricles are not communicating with each other. The atria send an impulse, but it is completely blocked at the AV node. Therefore impulses from the atria do not reach the ventricles, and the ventricles depend on their own inherent pacemaking capabilities (Figure 3-17).

Regularity. Rhythm is regular. The atria and ventricles are firing at their own rates and are completely independent of each other. Look at the PR interval; no correlation exists between the P waves and QRS complex—the key to this rhythm.

Rate. Atrial rate is between 60 and 100 bpm; ventricular rate is between 20 and 40 bpm.

P waves. Multiple P waves march along without any correlation to the QRS wave. P waves may be hidden in the QRS wave.

PRI. None.

QRS. Because the impulses are originating in the ventricles, the QRS wave may be greater than 0.12 seconds. If the pacemaking capability is originating in the junctional area, it may be less than 0.12 seconds.

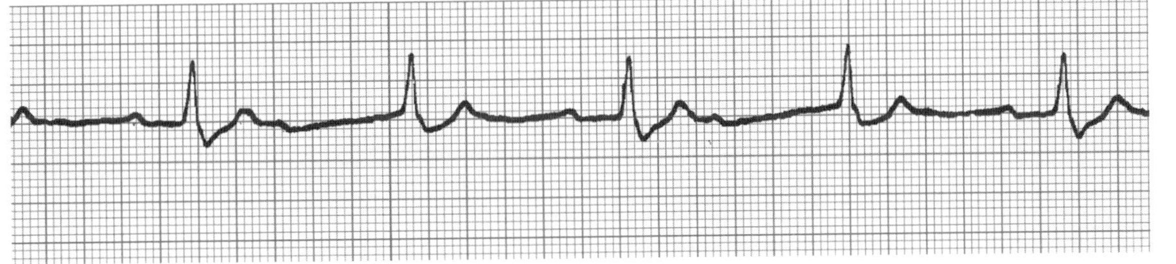

Figure 3-17 Third-degree (complete) heart block.

Premature ventricular contraction

There is always one unruly individual in every bunch. An irritable site in the ventricles refuses to accept that the SA node is in charge and occasionally speaks out of turn. An irritable focus in the ventricles prematurely fires, thereby causing an early beat (Figure 3-18). The key is a premature ventricular contraction (PVC) that is wide and a **T wave** that is usually in the opposite direction of the R wave.

Regularity. Rhythm is irregular because of the premature beats.

Rate. Rate is determined by the underlying rhythm.

P wave. P wave may be present, but it is likely to be dissociated.

PRI. None.

QRS. QRS wave is wide and bizarre and greater than 0.12 seconds.

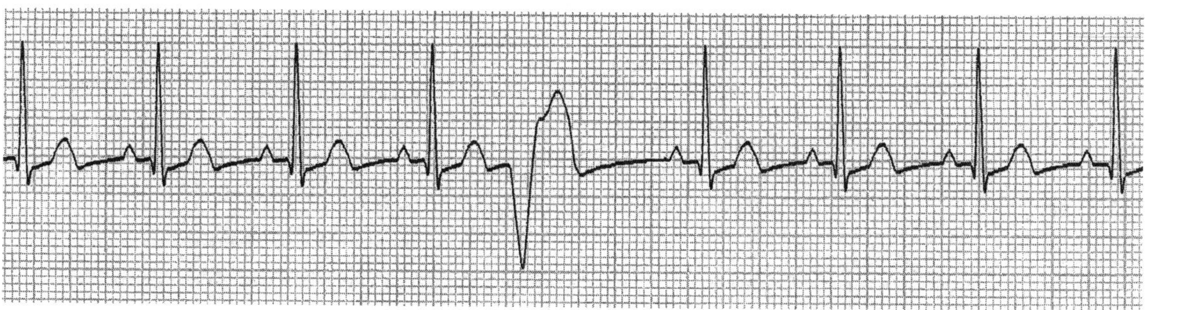

Figure 3-18 Premature ventricular contraction.

Ventricular tachycardia

Who said go? The ventricles have taken off and there is no catching them. An irritable focus in the ventricle is overriding the SA node. This focus may fire between 150 and 250 bpm (Figure 3-19). The ventricles are overriding the SA node because of an irritable focus in the ventricles.

Regularity. Rhythm is regular.

Rate. No atrial rate is measured; the ventricular rate is between 150 and 250 bpm.

P waves. None.

PRI. None.

QRS. Complex is greater than 0.12 seconds and originates in the ventricles.

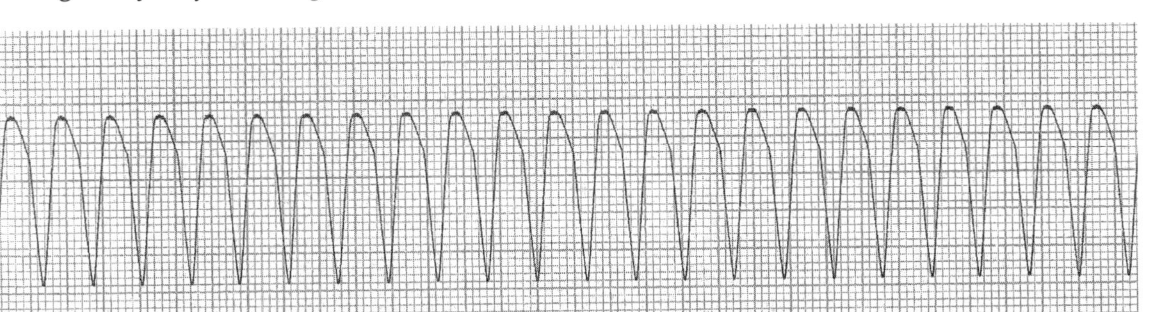

Figure 3-19 Ventricular tachycardia.

Ventricular fibrillation

Hold on a minute, you foci are all talking at the same time, and it's hard to keep a regular rhythm. Multiple foci in the ventricles fire at the same time (Figure 3-20).

Regularity. Rhythm is completely disorganized; no pattern is determined.

Rate. Rate cannot be determined because no noticeable complexes are observed.

P wave. None.

PRI. None.

QRS. None.

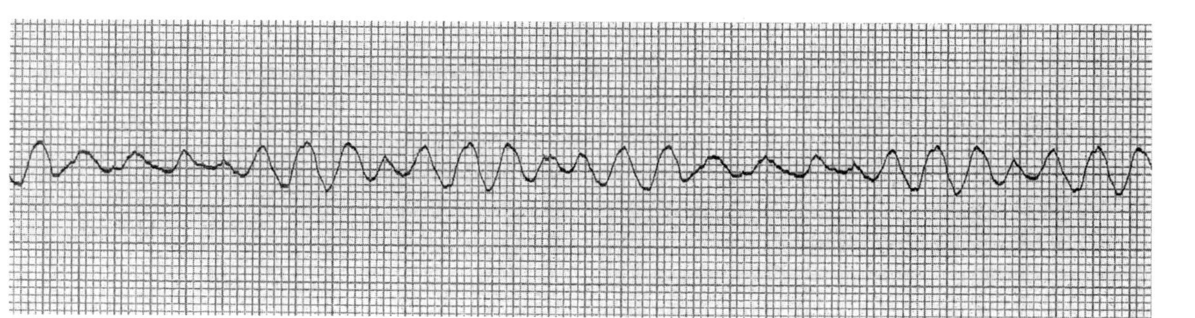

Figure 3-20 Ventricular fibrillation.

Idioventricular rhythm

Everyone is taking a break except the ventricles. The absence of a higher pacemaker causes the ventricles to initiate their own impulses. As you already know, the rate will be between 20 and 40 bpm (Figure 3-21). Nevertheless, the ventricles have a pacemaking capability at a rate of 20 to 40 bpm.

Regularity. Rhythm may be regular, depending on the firing capabilities.

Rate. Rate is between 20 and 40 bpm.

P-wave. No P waves. Impulse originates in the ventricles.

PRI. None.

QRS. QRS complex is greater than 0.12 seconds.

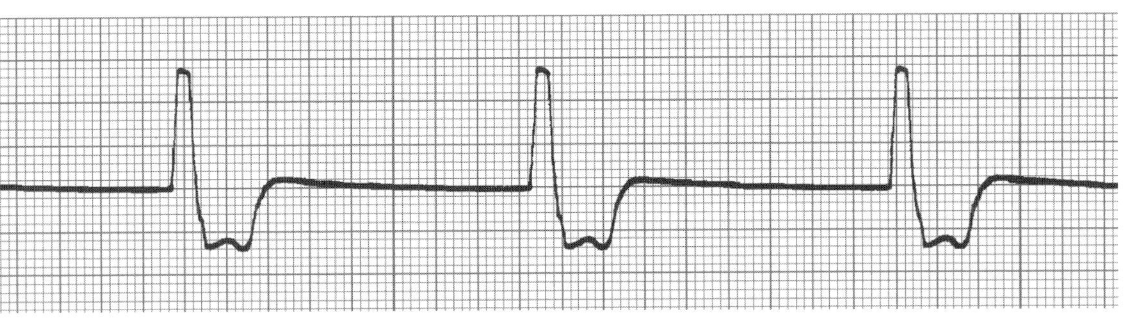

Figure 3-21 Idioventricular rhythm.

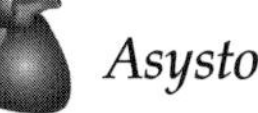 *Asystole*

Where did everyone go? No electrical activity is present. Complete absence of electrical rhythm (Figure 3-22).

Regularity. No complexes.
Rate. No complexes.
P wave. None.
PRI. None.
QRS. None.

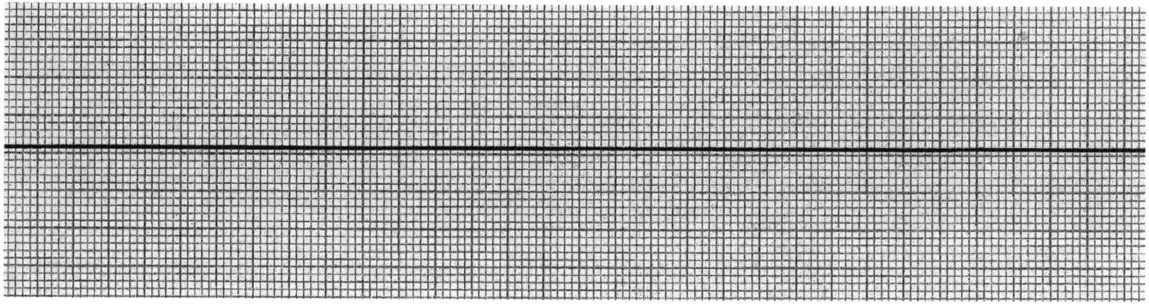

Figure 3-22 Asystole.

Vascular Access

Objectives

After completing this chapter, you will be able to:
1. *Define the listed key terms.*
2. *Identify intravenous solutions.*
3. *Describe the different intravenous catheters.*
4. *Discuss intraosseous infusion.*
5. *Discuss rectal medication administration.*
6. *Describe intravenous complications.*

Key Terms

Air embolism *Abnormal presence of air in the cardiovascular system. When air is introduced into the vein, an embolism may result, which can obstruct blood flow.*

Butterfly needle *Used for cannulating small veins, the butterfly needle has a winged appearance.*

Catheter shear *Teflon catheter that is introduced over the needle that may be inclined to shear once the catheter is advanced and then pulled back.*

Fluid overload *Excessive fluid accumulation in the body, which causes problems with circulation.*

Infection *Invasion of the body by germs that reproduce and multiply, causing disease by local cell injury, release of poisons, or germ antibody reaction in the cells. Infection may result at the intravenous site if poor aseptic technique is used.*

Infiltration *Fluid passing into tissues. Infiltration can result from IV cannulation.*

Macrodrip intravenous set *Device used to deliver large amounts of intravenous solution.*

Microdrip intravenous set *Device used to deliver small amounts of intravenous solution.*

Pyrogenic reactions *Reaction to bacteria that may cause shock, fever, headache, or backache.*

Thrombophlebitis *Inflammation of the vein accompanied by a clot. Prolonged intravenous therapy can cause thrombophlebitis.*

INTRODUCTION

Vascular access is an essential component of prehospital medicine and a component of the ALS Passport. It is used to gain access to the body's circulatory system. Vascular access is warranted when the need for medication administration exists or when fluid replacement is necessary. The basic provider may better assist with this procedure by understanding what IV equipment is needed during specific situations and by watching for potential complications. The companion CD-ROM to this text provides additional information on IV equipment.

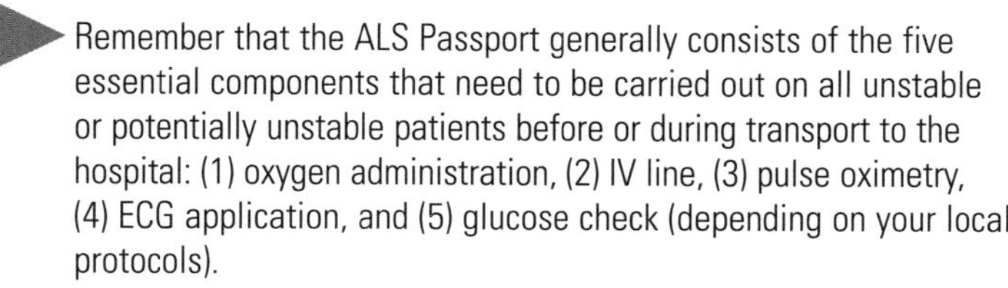

Remember that the ALS Passport generally consists of the five essential components that need to be carried out on all unstable or potentially unstable patients before or during transport to the hospital: (1) oxygen administration, (2) IV line, (3) pulse oximetry, (4) ECG application, and (5) glucose check (depending on your local protocols).

ADVANCED LIFE SUPPORT FOR BASIC LIFE SUPPORT PROCEDURES

INTRAVASCULAR ACCESS

Intravascular access is the procedure used to inject fluids, medication, or blood into a peripheral vein. Upper extremity veins are the preferred routes of choice, provided that the arms have no major injuries. Lower extremity veins may be used when upper extremity sites are inappropriate. The companion CD-ROM to this text provides additional information on intravascular access.

> Remember, during the intravascular access procedure, infiltration (the leaking of fluid into the subcutaneous tissues) can occur. When this happens, the IV should be discontinued. Prevention of fluid overflow is important and the reason you must provide continuous assessment of the patient's vital signs.

When will I see it?

- In unstable or potentially unstable patients
- When IV medication must be administered

When won't I see it?

- Stable patients who do not need IV medication

What should I watch for?

- Infection
- Pyrogenic reactions
- Infiltration
- Thrombophlebitis

- Fluid overload
- Air embolism
- Catheter shear
- Arterial puncture

Equipment

- $^1/_2$ or 1 inch adhesive tape.
- Alcohol and Betadine wipes.
- Butterfly needle (wing-type appearance).
- Commercial IV securing system.
- Constricting band.
- IV bag.
- IV catheters, sizes 14, 16, 18, 20, 22, or 24 gauge. The smaller the number, the larger the internal diameter of the IV catheter. If a patient is experiencing hypovolemia, a larger catheter (e.g., 14 or 16 gauge) is appropriate. Because the internal diameter of the catheter is larger, it allows for more volume to be infused. A smaller catheter (18 or 20 gauge) is appropriate for patients who do not need volume but who need a route for IV medication. In addition, a 22 gauge is appropriate for patients in the pediatric age group.
- IV solution with appropriate administration (microdrip or macrodrip set).
- Roller clamp.
- Sharps container.
- Vacutainer.

Preparation

- Examine all equipment, and check for defects (Figure 4-1).
- Double check the prescribed IV solution to ensure that it has not expired or that it is not cloudy or contaminated.

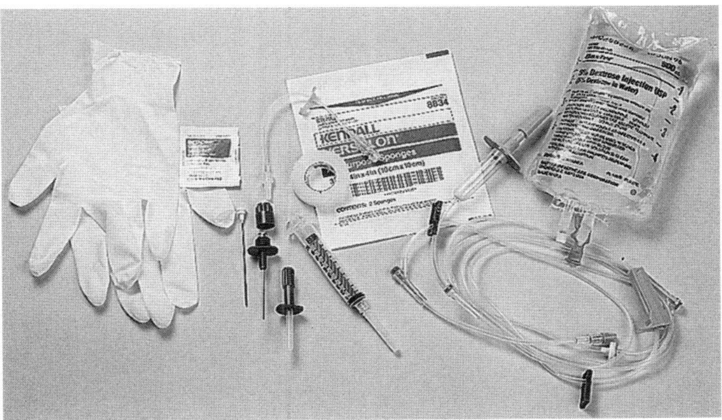

Figure 4-1 Equipment and supplies used to establish and maintain an intravenous line.

- Prepare the microdrip or macrodrip set, and attach it to the bag of solution.
- Prepare vacutainer syringe for blood aspiration, if needed.
- Cut or tear tape into several strips.
- Wear appropriate PPE: goggles, face shield, gloves, and gown. Both the advanced and basic providers should wear appropriate PPE.

Procedure summary

The basic provider should ask the advanced provider if an IV is necessary. He or she should gather all the appropriate equipment and assist the advanced provider with continuous patient assessment. The advanced provider inserts the IV catheter into a peripheral vein for fluid administration.

TYPES OF INTRAVASCULAR SOLUTIONS

5% Dextrose in water (D5W)

ACTIONS:	Glucose nutrient solution
INDICATIONS:	IV access for emergency drugs To dilute concentrated drugs for IV infusion
APPLICATIONS:	D_5W is used with a microdrip administration set of 60 drops (gtts)/mL and for general supportive care ([KVO] equals keep vein open or to keep open [TKO] equals 1 gtt every 3 seconds [10 gtts/min]).

0.9% Sodium chloride
(normal saline [NS] 250 mL/500 mL/1000 mL)

ACTIONS:	Fluid and sodium replacement
INDICATIONS:	Heat-related problems (e.g., heat exhaustion, heat stroke) Hypovolemia Diabetic ketoacidosis
APPLICATIONS:	9% sodium chloride is used with a microdrip administration set of 60 gtts/mL or macrodrip set of 10 gtts/mL or 15 gtts/mL and for either general supportive care or volume replacement (TKO or KVO).

Lactated Ringer's solution 1000 mL

ACTIONS:	Approximates the electrolyte concentration of the blood
INDICATIONS:	Hypovolemic shock
APPLICATIONS:	Lactated Ringer's solution is used with a macrodrip administration set of 15 gtts/mL, and for volume replacement. It may be used TKO or KVO.

Intravascular Access

Intravascular Access Steps

1. The advanced provider explains to the patient why the procedure is necessary and what it entails. The solution and administration set are prepared.

BLS Provider Steps

1. Prepare to:
   - Get the appropriate administration set (ask the advanced provider if he or she wants a microdrip or a macrodrip set).
   - Connect the IV tubing to the IV bag. The roller clamp on the IV tubing needs to be in the "off" position to avoid collecting air in the tubing and should be as close as possible to the IV bag. Once the clamp is off, you may squeeze the chamber in the tubing and allow it to fill to the midway point. There is a line that indicates how full the chamber needs to be. If the chamber fills up, the IV fluid will not flow. If this happens, flip the IV bag with the chamber upside down, squeeze the chamber to expel some of the fluid back into the IV bag, and clear up the IV chamber.
   - Open up the clamp once the chamber is filled to the appropriate level. Expel the air out of the tubing. You will see the IV fluid travel through the IV tubing. It is important to keep the end of the tubing (the part that goes into the IV catheter) as sterile as possible when opening to allow the air bubbles to escape the tubing. Once all the air bubbles are out, shut the clamp and make sure the cap is secure and covering the end of the tubing.

Continued

Intravascular Access—cont'd

Intravascular Access Steps

2. The advanced provider selects the appropriate catheter and prepares for cannulation.

3. The advanced provider cannulates the vein.

4. The IV solution is connected to the catheter.

5. The advanced provider secures the catheter in place.

6. The advanced provider reassesses the situation.

BLS Provider Steps

2. Prepare to:
   - Retrieve the requested catheter, alcohol wipes, 1/2 or 1 inch tape or a commercial IV securing system, and constricting band.
   - Cleanse the site.
3. Prepare to:
   - Give the advanced provider equipment as requested.
   - Ensure that all sharps are disposed of in the appropriate container.
4. Prepare to:
   - Hand the line to the advanced provider.
   - Set the drip rate as requested. It could be set to the KVO or TKO rate.
   - Watch the chamber; set the flow for about 10 gtt/min. The drops entering the chamber can be adjusted with the roller clamp on the IV tubing.
5. Hand the advanced provider the strips of tape to secure the catheter. If requested, tape it to the IV.
6. Watch for infiltration (hematoma) or discoloration around the IV site. Infiltration indicates that the vein has ruptured and that fluid is leaking into the surrounding tissues. Discoloration around the IV indicates the possibility of an allergic response or ecchymosis from the IV puncture into the vein.

On the Scene

You are on the scene with a patient who is complaining of chest pain. She is conscious and alert. The patient's vital signs are blood pressure 160/88, heart rate 88, and respiratory rate 22, and she is cool and clammy. The patient is receiving oxygen via a nonrebreather mask, and the ECG monitor and pulse oximeter have been applied. The advanced provider would like to prepare for IV cannulation. You gather an IV bag and administration set, alcohol wipes, constricting band, 18 or 20 gauge catheter (the patient is not hypovolemic), and tape to secure the IV to the patient. The IV is initiated and secured. You further assist by watching for infiltration, a nonflowing IV, or fluid overload, which may result in pulmonary edema or hypertension.

INTRAOSSEOUS INFUSION

Intraosseous (IO) infusion is the injection of fluids, medication, or blood into bone marrow rather than into a vein (Figure 4-2). The technique of IO needle placement is simple, quick, and safe. It is usually used for the rapid administration of fluid in the critically ill or injured pediatric patient. All resuscitation drugs may be effectively delivered through an IO needle. IO infusion requires a heavy-gauge needle with a stylet. The stylet is used to prevent plugging when advanced through the bone before entering the marrow space. The anterior tibia just below the knee is the site of insertion. Gaining IV access on a pediatric patient who is experiencing cardiopulmonary arrest does not warrant prolonged attempts in the field. If an IV site cannot be obtained within 90 seconds, an IO infusion needs to be considered. However, if the patient is intubated, remember that some medications may be administered through the ET tube. The companion CD-ROM to this text provides additional information on intraosseous infusion.

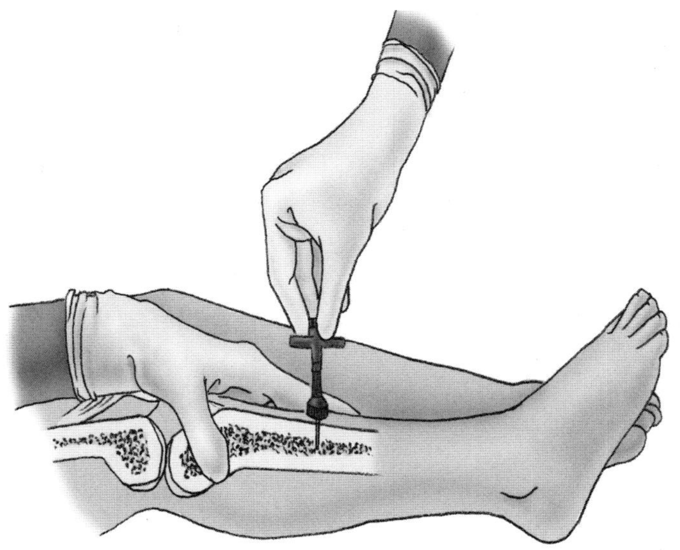

Figure 4-2 Intraosseous infusion.

When will I see it?

- Attempts to establish a peripheral IV have failed.
- Fluid and drug resuscitation is necessary for the child who is unconscious, unresponsive, or in danger of dying.
- Sternal IO infusion is applicable for adult patients.

When won't I see it?

- Fracture above the insertion site is absolutely contraindicated.
- Infection or burn at the site, unless no other options are appropriate.

What should I watch for?

- Infiltration
- Obstruction

Equipment

- 1 inch tape
- 10 mL syringe
- 4 to 6 mL of NS
- 4 × 4 gauze pads
- Alcohol and Betadine wipes
- Antibiotic ointment
- Extension tubing (optional)
- IO needle
- IV solution and administration (microdrip or macrodrip) set
- Sharps container

Preparation

- Examine all equipment, and check for defects.
- Check the IV bag for cloudiness, and squeeze it for leaks.
- Prepare the microdrip or macrodrip administration set, and attach it to the bag of solution.
- Wear appropriate PPE: goggles, face shield, gloves, and gown. Both the advanced and basic providers should wear appropriate PPE.

Procedure summary

The advanced provider inserts the IO needle into the bone marrow and withdraws the stylet. The advanced provider attaches the 10 mL syringe to the IO needle, inserts 3 mL of NS, and then aspirates. If blood and marrow is observed in the syringe after aspiration, then the IO needle is in the marrow cavity.

Intraosseous Infusion

Intraosseous Infusion Steps

1. The advanced provider explains the procedure and what it entails to the patient.

2. The advanced provider inserts the needle until it penetrates the bone marrow. The stylet is removed. Bone marrow is aspirated into the saline-filled syringe. Placement is ensured.

3. The needle is secured.

BLS Provider Steps

1. Prepare to:
   - Cleanse the site of cannulation.
   - Open the IV bag envelope at the edge where it is notched.
   - Read the name of the solution to the advanced provider.
   - Open the IV tubing and extension tubing (optional), connecting all pieces of tubing together.
   - Close the roller clamp below the drip chamber.
   - Insert the IV tubing in the IV solution bag portal.
   - Squeeze the drip chamber until it is half full of solution.
   - Uncap the distal end of tubing while preventing contamination of cap.
   - Open the valve flow solution until all bubbles are out.
   - Close the tubing valve, and recap the distal end of the tube.

2. Retrieve the IO needle and 10 mL syringe with 6 mL of NS.

3. Be prepared to:
   - Secure the needle with the 4 × 4 gauze pad. Tape the needle as if it was an impaled object.
   - Watch for infiltration, dislodgment of the needle, fluid overload, and poor flowing IV solution.

On the Scene

You are on the scene with a pediatric patient in cardiac arrest. The patient has been intubated. However, as a result of vascular collapse, starting an IV line is difficult. The advanced provider requests the preparation for IO insertion. You gather an IO needle, a 10 mL syringe filled with 6 mL of NS, IV bag with administration set, alcohol wipes, 4 × 4 gauze, and tape. The advanced provider finds the appropriate landmark (2 to 3 finger widths below and medial to the knee) and inserts the needle. The stylet from within the needle is removed and disposed of appropriately. The advanced provider attaches a 10 mL syringe to the needle, inserts approximately 3 mL of NS and then aspirates to confirm proper placement in the bone marrow. On aspiration, blood and bone marrow may not be noticed in the syringe. Once appropriate placement of the IO needle is confirmed, you attach the IV tubing to the needle and assist in securing the needle to the leg. You further assist by watching for infiltration, nonflowing IV (no drops are noted in the IV chamber), or fluid overload, which may result in pulmonary edema or hypertension.

Pharmacology and Medication Administration

5

Objectives

After completing this chapter, you will be able to:
1. *Define the listed key terms.*
2. *Name common medications used in the prehospital setting.*

Key Terms

Acetylcholine *Type of neurotransmitter that stimulates the parasympathetic nervous system.*

Acidosis *Abnormal increase of hydrogen ions (acid) in the blood.*

Antidysrhythmic *Medication used to suppress cardiac dysrhythmias.*

Bronchodilator *Agent that causes relaxation (widening) of the bronchial smooth muscle, thereby improving airflow.*

Chronotrope *Substance that affects heart rate. A positive chronotrope increases heart rate, whereas a negative chronotrope decreases it.*

Diuresis *Increases urine secretion.*

Dysrhythmia *Any cardiac rhythm other than a normal sinus rhythm.*

Hemodynamically unstable *Unstable vital signs.*

Inotrope *Substance that improves the contractility of a muscle, particularly the heart.*

Parasympatholytic *Blocks the action of the parasympathetic nervous system.*
Status epilepticus *Recurrent generalized seizure during which no resumption of consciousness occurs; a seizure that lasts longer than 15 minutes.*
Sympathomimetic *Mimics or stimulates the sympathetic nervous system.*
Urticaria *Skin reaction that is characterized by a rash and accompanied by itching.*

INTRODUCTION

This chapter is designed to be used only as a reference and not as a protocol or authorization to use medication. It will help you become familiar with medications used in the pre-hospital environment. As a basic provider, you can assist the advanced provider by knowing how medications are packaged, where they are located, how to assemble them, and where to check for expiration dates. Everyone should use a double-check system. Before administering, a drug should be checked to ensure that is the correct type, that it has not expired, and that it is not cloudy or solidified. Medications come in a variety of delivery systems. Familiarity with the equipment needed with each delivery system helps avoid delays in administration.

MEDICATION PACKAGING

As a basic provider you should become familiar with the packaging of the various types of medications used in your system and where they are located. Medications that are used in the emergency setting are typically found in pre-filled syringes, ampules, or vials, or mixed in an IV solution. The companion CD-ROM to this text provides additional information on packaging.

MEDICATION ADMINISTRATION

Medications may be administered via the ET or IO route; IV, subcutaneous (SQ), or intramuscular (IM) injection; inhalation, or rectally. The companion CD-ROM to this text provides additional information on medication administration.

ADVANCED LIFE SUPPORT FOR BASIC LIFE SUPPORT PROCEDURES

NEBULIZER TREATMENT

A nebulizer is used to administer medication via inhalation. Nebulized medication is generally used to treat bronchospasms in respiratory disorders, such as asthma or chronic obstructive pulmonary disease (Figure 5-1). The companion CD-ROM to this text provides additional information on nebulizer treatment.

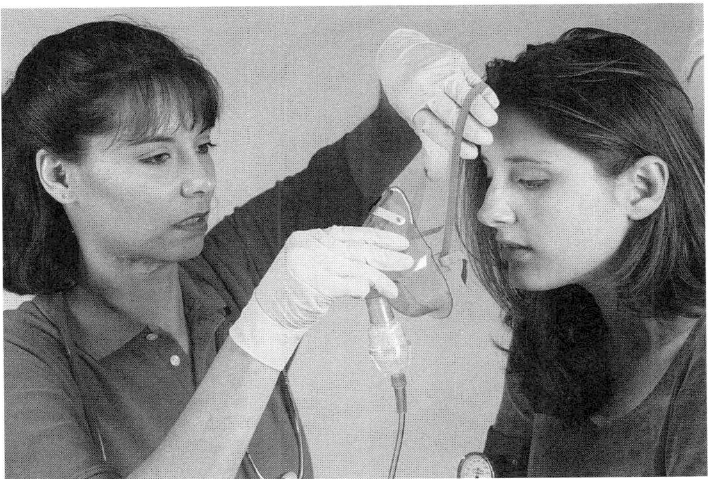

Figure 5-1 Nebulizer treatment.

When will I see it?

- Patient has minimum-to-moderate difficulty breathing because of bronchospasm.

When won't I see it?

- Patient is unable to inhale the drug because of severe bronchospasm.
- Bronchodilation is not warranted.

What should I watch for?

- Patient tires from the work of breathing.
- Increased heart rate is measured.
- Poor inhalation of the medication is the result of patient talking or moving.
- No misting is noted from the breathing tube as a result of low flow of oxygen (prevents medication uptake into the nebulizing chamber).

Equipment

- Aerosol face mask.
- Bronchodilation medication.
- Mouthpiece.
- Nebulizer.
- Nebulizing chamber.
- Oxygen supply tubing.
- Oxygen with a flow meter set at 6 to 8 L per minute (L/min). A minimum of 700 psi is needed in the oxygen tank for adequate flow.
- Stopwatch.
- T-piece.

Preparation

- Examine all equipment, and check for defects.
- Check the expiration date for each prescribed medication. Ensure that the solution is clear (not cloudy) and not contaminated.

- Wear appropriate PPE: goggles, face shield, gloves, and gown. Both the advanced and basic providers should wear appropriate PPE.

Procedure summary

The nebulizer needs to be assembled, and the basic provider should be familiar with the assembly steps. Once assembled, the basic provider should alert the advanced provider that the nebulizer is ready. The advanced provider will then insert the desired medication. If the patient is too exhausted to hold the nebulizer, the basic provider may have to connect the nebulizer to a nebulizing mask.

Nebulizer Treatment

Nebulizer Treatment Steps	BLS Provider Steps
1. The advanced provider prepares the prescribed medication.	1. Retrieve medication and connect the following: • Oxygen supply tubing to the nebulizer • T-piece to the top of the nebulizing chamber • Mouthpiece to the T-piece. (Note: If patient is unable to use mouthpiece, use an aerosol mask.) • Oxygen supply tubing to the oxygen flowmeter
2. The advanced provider instructs and gives nebulizer treatment to the patient.	2. Be prepared to: • Set the oxygen flowmeter to 6 L/min, which is usually sufficient to avoid wasting medication. However, if an aerosol mask is used, the flowmeter is set to 10 L/min. • Confirm that the medication is misting out from the end of the tubing.

Continued

Nebulizer Treatment—cont'd

Nebulizer Treatment Steps	BLS Provider Steps
3. The advanced provider assists the patient as required.	3. If the patient is unable to hold the nebulizer: • Remove the mouthpiece from the T-piece. • Take a simple mask, and remove the oxygen tubing from the mask. • Insert the T-piece into the mask. Apply the mask to the patient. • Be aware that these patients are very sick and may need ventilatory assistance.
4. The advanced provider reassesses the patient.	4. Be prepared to: • Auscultate the patient's lungs to confirm whether more air entry and less wheezing have occurred. • Monitor the heart rate. You should notify the advanced provider if the rate goes above 150 bpm. • Monitor blood pressure throughout the treatment. • Monitor respiratory status (rate and depth) frequently. • Apply a nasal cannula to increase oxygen concentration during the treatment, if necessary.

RECTAL MEDICATION ADMINISTRATION

In some emergency cases the administration of a medication may be administered rectally. Diazapam (Valium) is the most common drug to be administered in this manner, and it may be used in the pediatric age group for seizure management. Rectal administration may also be used to medicate adults.

When will I see it?

- IV access cannot be established.
- Patient has persistent seizure activity.

When won't I see it?

- When IV access has been established.

What should I watch for?

- Protecting the patient from injury if a seizure is present.
- Patient is not responding to rectal administration of anti-seizure medication. Attempts to establish IV access should continue.

Equipment

- 3 mL syringe
- 14 or 16 gauge catheter (catheter ONLY, no needle)
- Sharps container
- Medication

Preparation

- Wear appropriate PPE: goggles, face shield, gloves, and gown. Both the advanced and basic providers should wear appropriate PPE.

Rectal Medication Administration

Rectal Medication Administration Steps	BLS Provider Steps
1. The advanced provider inserts a catheter into the rectal mucosa and administers the medication.	1. Prepare to: • Retrieve a 14 or 16 gauge catheter. • Separate the buttocks. • Protect the patient from injury if the patient is actively seizing.

On the Scene

You are on the scene with a patient who is experiencing an acute asthma attack. The patient's vital signs are blood pressure 156/90, heart rate 110, and respiratory rate 28. Wheezes are noted bilaterally on exhalation. The patient is placed on oxygen, an IV is initiated, and the ECG monitor and pulse oximeter have been attached to the patient. The advanced provider requests a nebulizer treatment for the patient. You assist by gathering oxygen supply tubing, a nebulizing chamber, T-piece, mouthpiece, and oxygen with a flow meter. You also assist by retrieving the medication and double checking it with the advanced provider. Once the nebulizer is assembled, the flow meter is set between 6 and 8 L/min or 6 and 10 L/min if a face mask is used. The patient is then allowed to inhale the medication.

DRAWING BLOOD

Blood should be drawn from every patient who has an altered level of consciousness or chest pain, or from any patient the advanced provider believes is necessary (Figure 5-2). The advanced provider may choose to draw blood in many other situations, and the basic provider may assist by knowing what equipment is needed.

When will I see it?

- Altered mental status
- History of diabetes
- Overdose
- Chest pain

When won't I see it?

- Blood may be drawn at the discretion of the advanced provider.

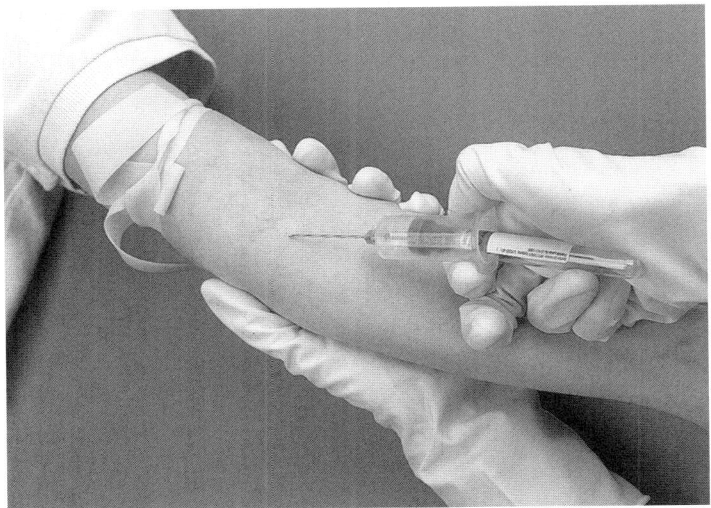

Figure 5-2 Obtaining a blood sample with a vacutainer.

What should I watch for?

- Hematoma
- Very little or no blood collecting in the vacutainer
- Removal of constricting band after completion of the procedure

Equipment

- 18 or 20 gauge needle
- Alcohol wipes
- Blood tubes
- Constricting band
- IV catheter
- Label
- Sharps container
- Vacutainer
- Writing utensil

Preparation

- Prepare all equipment in advance.
- Wear appropriate PPE: goggles, face shield, gloves, and gown. Both the advanced and basic providers should wear appropriate PPE.

Drawing Blood

Drawing Blood Steps	BLS Provider Steps
1. The advanced provider uses a vacutainer to withdraw the specific amount of blood required per protocol.	1. Prepare to label the patient's blood tube with the following: • Time it was drawn • Name of the provider who drew the blood • Patient's name • Date

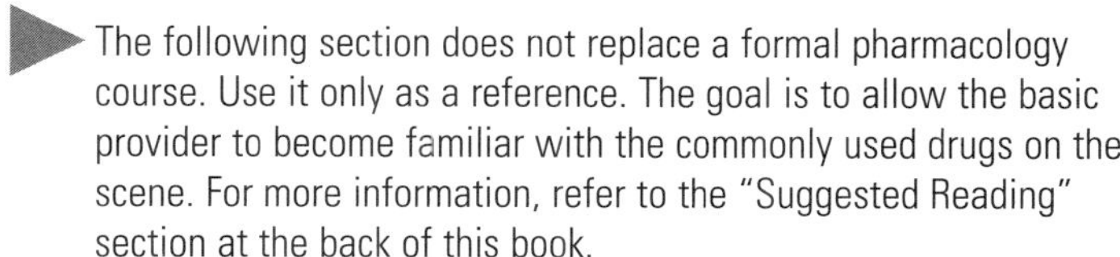
The following section does not replace a formal pharmacology course. Use it only as a reference. The goal is to allow the basic provider to become familiar with the commonly used drugs on the scene. For more information, refer to the "Suggested Reading" section at the back of this book.

PHARMACOLOGY TABLE

Amiodarone (Cordarone)

ACTIONS:	Antidysrhythmic substance
INDICATIONS:	Ventricular fibrillation
	Hemodynamically unstable ventricular tachycardia
	Paroxysmal supraventricular tachycardia
APPLICATIONS:	Amiodarone is an antidysrhythmic medication used to treat atrial and ventricular dysrhythmias. Amiodarone is used more routinely in the hospital setting. However, it may also be used in the prehospital setting.

Aspirin

ACTIONS:	Analgesic substance
	Antiinflammatory medication
	Antipyretic (fever-reducing) drug
	Antiplatelet medication
INDICATIONS:	Mild-to-moderate pain or fever
	To prevent platelet aggregation in ischemia
	Thromboembolism
	Unstable angina
	To prevent myocardial infarction or reinfarction

Atropine

ACTIONS:	Blocks acetylcholine receptors
	Positive chronotrope (increases heart rate)
	Decreases gastrointestinal secretions
INDICATIONS:	Bradycardia
	Hypotension secondary to bradycardia
	Asystole
	Organophosphate poisoning
APPLICATIONS:	Atropine is a parasympatholytic substance, which means it blocks the parasympathetic system, thereby allowing the sympathetic system to take over and increase the heart rate.

50% Dextrose

ACTIONS:	To rapidly elevate blood glucose level
INDICATIONS:	Hypoglycemia
APPLICATIONS:	Glucose is used when managing a patient with hypoglycemia. The normal glucose level range is between 90 and 120 mg/dL. However, you should treat the patient and not the glucometer. Remember, 50% dextrose is water with 25 g sugar. This medication is administered to patients who are hypoglycemic, to those with a glucose level <60 mg/dL, and to patients with signs and symptoms of hypoglycemia.

Diazapam (Valium)

ACTIONS:	Anticonvulsant
	Skeletal muscle relaxant
	Sedative
INDICATIONS:	Major motor seizures
	Status epilepticus
	Premedication before cardioversion
	Skeletal muscle relaxant
	Acute anxiety states

Diazapam (Valium)—cont'd
   APPLICATIONS: Diazapam is a controlled substance. Therefore only an advanced level provider has access to it. Diazapam has multiple uses, primarily for seizure control.

Diphenhydramine (Benadryl)
   ACTIONS: Blocks histamine receptors
      Sedative
   INDICATIONS: Anaphylaxis
      Allergic reactions
   APPLICATIONS: When a foreign substance is introduced into the body, it may be rejected. When the body rejects a substance, it breaks down certain cells, which releases histamine. Histamine is a potent chemical that causes bronchoconstriction, urticaria, increased vascular permeability, and hypotension. Diphenhydramine blocks the release of histamine and helps prevent further complications.

Dopamine (Intropin)
   ACTIONS: Positive inotrope (increases force of contractions)
      Positive chronotrope (increases heart rate)
      Selectively dilates blood vessels of the kidney, gastrointestinal system, brain, and heart
   INDICATIONS: Cardiogenic shock
      Hypovolemic shock (only after complete fluid resuscitation)

Continued

Dopamine (Intropin)—cont'd

APPLICATIONS: When a patient is experiencing hypotension and the cause is not related to hypovolemia or bradycardia, dopamine is considered. Dopamine is a vasoconstrictor; it helps constrict the vessels, which cause the blood pressure to increase.

Epinephrine 1:1000

ACTIONS: Bronchodilator
Positive chronotrope (increases heart rate)
Positive inotrope (increases force of heart contraction)

INDICATIONS: Bronchial asthma
Exacerbation of some forms of chronic obstructive pulmonary disease
Anaphylaxis

Epinephrine 1:10,000

ACTIONS: Positive chronotrope (increases heart rate)
Positive inotrope (increases outflow of blood with each heart contraction)
Causes bronchodilation

INDICATIONS: Ventricular fibrillation
Pulseless ventricular tachycardia
Asystole
Patients with pulseless electrical activity (PEA) displayed on the cardiac monitor (patients with PEA get epinephrine)

APPLICATIONS: The size of the syringe or vial may distinguish epinephrine 1:1000 from 1:10,000, depending on how the

Epinephrine 1:10,000—cont'd

medication is packaged. Epinephrine 1:10,000 contains more fluid, therefore it is contained in a larger syringe; 1:1000 means 1 milligram of the medication in 1 milliliter of fluid, and 1:10,000 means 1 milligram of medication in 10 milliliters of fluid. Epinephrine is a sympathomimetic substance because it mimics the response of the sympathetic system.

Furosemide (Lasix)

ACTIONS: Inhibits reabsorption of sodium chloride
Promotes prompt diuresis
Vasodilation

INDICATIONS: Congestive heart failure
Pulmonary edema

APPLICATIONS: Furosemide is used when excess fluid needs to be removed, such as in congestive heart failure.

Lidocaine

ACTIONS: Suppresses ventricular ectopic activity
Increases ventricular fibrillation threshold
Reduces velocity of electrical impulses through conductive system

INDICATIONS: Malignant PVCs
Ventricular tachycardia
Ventricular fibrillation

APPLICATIONS: If the ventricles become irritable, causing an irregular rhythm, lidocaine is used to "soothe" the ventricles and help eliminate any irritability.

Albuterol (Proventil)

ACTIONS:	Bronchodilator Relieves bronchospasms
INDICATIONS:	Bronchial asthma Reversible bronchospasm associated with chronic bronchitis and emphysema
APPLICATIONS:	Commonly used bronchodilator that helps relieve bronchospasm.

L-Albuterol (Xopenex)

Action:	Bronchodilator Relieves bronchospasms
INDICATIONS:	Bronchial asthma Reversible bronchospasm associated with chronic bronchitis and emphysema
APPLICATIONS:	New bronchodilator that helps relieve bronchospasm with less cardiac side effects than Albuterol

Morphine sulfate

ACTIONS:	Central nervous system depressant Causes peripheral vasodilation Decreases sensitivity to pain
INDICATIONS:	Severe pain Pulmonary edema
APPLICATIONS:	Morphine is a controlled medication used to relieve pain and anxiety. Morphine is typically used with the patient who is having chest pain to help alleviate discomfort. If the discomfort is alleviated, the heart will work less and the need for extra blood flow will decrease.

Naloxone (Narcan)

ACTIONS:	Reverses effects of narcotics
INDICATIONS:	Narcotic overdoses including morphine, Demerol, heroin, Dilaudid, Paregoric, Percodan, fentanyl, and methadone
	Synthetic analgesic overdoses including Nubain, Talwin, Stadol, and Darvon
	Alcoholic coma
	To rule out narcotics in coma of unknown origin
APPLICATIONS:	Naloxone will typically be administered to all unconscious and unresponsive patients. It is used to reverse the effects of narcotics.

Nitroglycerin spray or tablets

ACTIONS:	Dilates coronary arteries
	Dilates systemic arteries
INDICATIONS:	Angina pectoris
	Chest pain associated with myocardial infarction
APPLICATIONS:	Blood pressure levels must be checked before and after nitroglycerin is administered. Nitroglycerin causes vasodilation and will drop the patient's blood pressure. The patient may also experience a headache as a result of the vasodilation. You should not touch the tablets or inhale the spray while assisting with the administration of this medication. The nitroglycerin tablet is placed under the patient's tongue. With nitroglycerin spray, the patient is asked to hold his or her breath and to touch the roof of his or her mouth with the tongue before placing the medication under

Continued

Nitroglycerin spray or tablets—cont'd

the tongue. It is important to inquire whether the patient is taking Viagra before administration; together, these two medications may have a detrimental effect such as severe hypotension.

Sodium bicarbonate

ACTIONS:
Combines with excessive acids to form a weak volatile acid

Reduces the acidic state of the blood

INDICATIONS:
Metabolic acidosis as determined by arterial blood gas studies

Tricyclic antidepressant overdoses

APPLICATIONS:
There are two types of acidosis: (1) respiratory acidosis, which is caused by a respiratory problem; and (2) metabolic acidosis, which is caused by a metabolic problem. A lack of oxygen and a build up of carbon dioxide in the body causes respiratory acidosis; it needs to be treated with oxygen. Diabetic ketoacidosis (DKA) or aspirin overdose may also cause metabolic acidosis. It may be treated with sodium bicarbonate.

Adenosine (Adenocard)

ACTIONS:
Slows supraventricular tachycardia

INDICATIONS:
Supraventricular tachycardia

APPLICATIONS:
Adenosine is used to treat supraventricular tachycardia. However, the administration of this medication is a little scary for the practitioner, because it might cause a short burst of asystole shortly after the administration.

Adenosine (Adenocard)—cont'd

| | The asystole occurs for only a brief period, and the patient should be watched carefully. |

Vasopressin (Pitressin)

ACTIONS: Nonadrenergic vasoconstrictor

INDICATIONS: Alternative to epinephrine in ventricular fibrillation

APPLICATIONS: Vasopressin is a vasoconstrictor that is used as a one-time dose in ventricular fibrillation. The benefits of vasopressin last longer than the benefits of epinephrine, thus its advantage, and it is able to work more effectively in acidotic conditions.

Midazolam (Versed)

ACTIONS: Anticonvulsant
Skeletal muscle relaxant
Sedative

INDICATIONS: Major motor seizures
Status epilepticus
Premedication before cardioversion

APPLICATIONS: Midazolam is a controlled substance, therefore only the advanced practitioner will have access to it.

Etomidate (Amidate)

ACTIONS: Sedative

INDICATIONS: Preintubation sedative
Premedication before cardioversion

APPLICATIONS: Etomidate is a rapid-acting sedative used in the prehospital setting to assist intubation and to sedate the patient before cardioversion.

Gadgets

6

Objectives

After completing this chapter, you will be able to:
1. *Define the listed key terms.*
2. *Explain the purpose of a glucose check and how to perform the procedure.*
3. *Explain the purpose of a pulse oximeter and how to apply it.*
4. *Explain the importance of the end-tidal carbon dioxide detector and how to use it.*

Key Terms

Anemia *Decreased hemoglobin level in the blood.*
Glucometer *Small machine that calculates and displays the patient's glucose reading.*
Lancet *Short, pointed blade used to obtain a drop of blood.*

ADVANCED LIFE SUPPORT FOR BASIC LIFE SUPPORT PROCEDURES

GLUCOSE MONITORING

Glucose monitoring is an essential component of prehospital management and a component of the ALS Passport. Glucose monitoring should be considered in all patients, especially in those who are unconscious or exhibit an altered mental status. Glucose monitoring is the determination of the level of glucose in the blood. There are several ways to determine this level, therefore it is important that you are familiar with your system or with the method recommended by your department or state.

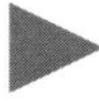 Remember, the ALS Passport generally consists of the five essential components that need to be carried out on all unstable or potentially unstable patients before or during transport to the hospital: (1) oxygen administration, (2) IV line, (3) pulse oximetry, (4) ECG application, and (5) glucose check (depending on your local protocols).

When will I see it?

Patients experiencing any of the following conditions should have their glucose level checked:

- Altered mental status
- Weakness
- Syncope
- Dizziness
- Cardiac arrest
- Diabetes

When won't I see it?

- It should be considered for every patient.

What should I watch for?

- Glucose reading <60 mg/dL
- Glucose reading >120 mg/dL

Equipment

- Alcohol wipes
- Lancet or small needle
- Glucometer (Figure 6-1)
- Glucose strip or stick
- Sharps container

Preparation

- Examine all equipment, and check for defects.
- Wear appropriate PPE: goggles, face shield, gloves, and gown. Both the advanced and basic providers should wear appropriate PPE.

Procedure summary

Depending on your system or local protocol, you may be expected to assist with this procedure or to perform it yourself.

 Remember, a normal glucose reading is between 90 and 120 mg/dL.

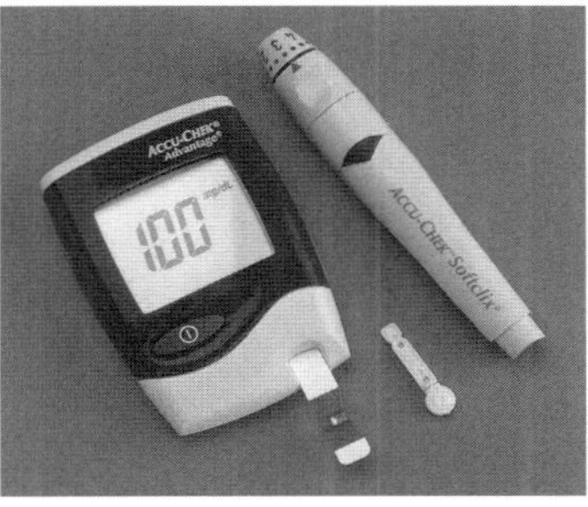

Figure 6-1 Glucometer.

Glucose Monitoring

Glucose Monitoring Steps	BLS Provider Steps
1. The advanced provider prepares the patient for drawing a blood sample.	1. Prepare to: • Gather alcohol wipes and a lancet. (A small needle may be used instead of a lancet.) • Set the lancet in the glucose monitoring device. • Ensure that the glucose stick matches the glucometer. • Turn on the glucometer.
2. The advanced provider will prick the patient's finger and place a drop of blood on the glucose stick. The measurement is taken.	2. Be prepared to: • Place the drop of blood on the appropriate side of the stick. • Place the glucose stick inside the glucometer. Wait for a reading, which may take up to 60 seconds, depending on the monitor being used.

PULSE OXIMETER

Pulse oximetry is an essential component of prehospital management and a component of the ALS Passport. The pulse oximeter is a device used to monitor oxygen saturation, and it should be used on all unstable or potentially unstable patients. The device determines the level of oxygen present in the red blood cells and should be used as part of a baseline patient assessment. Its reading represents a value called *percentage saturation.* Normally, blood has a partial pressure of oxygen in the artery (PaO_2) of 90 to 100 mm Hg, with a corresponding oxygen saturation of between 97% and 99%. When the PaO_2 falls below 60 mm Hg, the oxygen saturation measured by pulse oximetry generally reads less than 90%. Thus even when the oxygen saturation remains above 90%, the actual carrying capacity of the blood or the percentage of red blood cells carrying oxygen may have decreased by as much as 40%. It is important to note that the pulse oximeter is only an indirect measure of oxygen saturation of red blood cells, based on light absorption by red blood cells. For this reason, it is important that the saturation reading be kept relatively high and between 95% and 100%. The pulse oximeter may give an inaccurate reading when:

- Nail polish is on the nail bed.
- Dirt is on the nail bed.
- Patient is hypothermic.
- Patient is hypovolemic.
- Carbon monoxide present in the blood.
- Patient is anemic.

Advantages:

- Rapid access to patient oxygen saturation

When will I see it?

- Unstable or potentially unstable patients
- Patients who may have an underlying oxygen/carbon dioxide compromise

When won't I see it?

- Patients who are stable and do not require continuous monitoring

What should I look for?

- Drop in oxygen saturation less than 94%

Equipment

- Pulse oximeter
- Finger or ear lobe clip

Preparation

- Examine all equipment, and check for defects.
- Wear appropriate PPE: goggles, face shield, gloves, and gown. Both the advanced and basic providers should wear appropriate PPE.

Procedure summary

The pulse oximeter is attached to the ear lobe or finger, depending on which clip is used. Typically, the pulse oximeter is attached to the patient's finger, over the nail bed (Figure 6-2). Once the pulse oximeter is turned on, the advanced provider ensures that the heart rate displayed corresponds to the patient's pulse rate and records the reading.

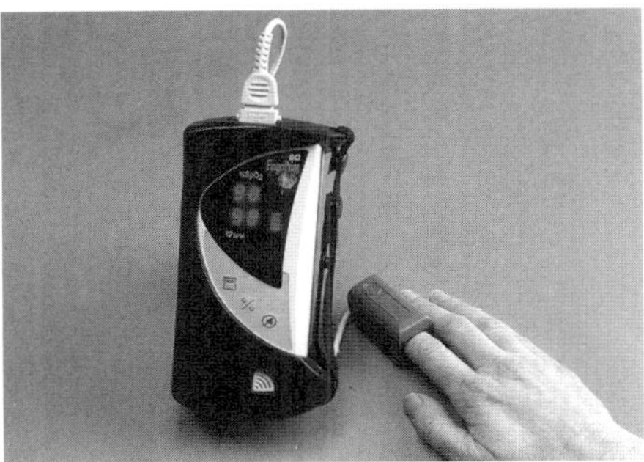

Figure 6-2 Pulse oximeter.

Pulse Oximeter

BLS Provider Steps

1. Ensure that the patient's nail bed is clean of debris and nail polish.
2. Attach the pulse oximeter clip to the patient's finger, covering the nail bed.
3. Turn on the monitor.

END-TIDAL CARBON DIOXIDE MONITORING

The end-tidal carbon dioxide detector helps determine whether the ET tube is correctly placed in the trachea rather than inadvertently placed in the esophagus. An end-tidal carbon dioxide detector should be used in conjunction with the assessment of breath sounds, evidence of improving perfusion, bilateral symmetrical chest rise, and use of pulse oximetry to confirm ET tube placement.

Some devices identify carbon dioxide levels by a color change. If the ET tube is in the trachea, the color in the end-tidal carbon dioxide detector turns yellow to indicate the passage of carbon dioxide during exhalation (YELLOW for YES). If the ET tube is placed in the esophagus, the color within the detector remains purple (PURPLE for POOR), indicating a lack of carbon dioxide (Figure 6-3). Other devices give a digital read-out of the estimated end-tidal carbon dioxide. A normal end-tidal carbon dioxide valve is generally 35 to 45 mm Hg.

When will I see it?

• When used in conjunction with ET tube ventilation.

When won't I see it?

• When an ET tube is not used.

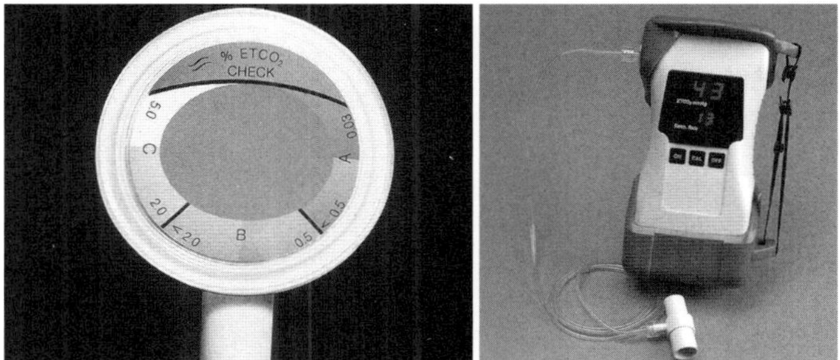

Figure 6-3 End-tidal carbon dioxide detectors.

What should I watch for?

- Watch for a change in color in the device after exhalation. If the color does not change but remains purple, the ET tube may be inserted in the esophagus. If the color within the detector changes to yellow, carbon dioxide is detected after exhalation and the ET tube is placed in the trachea. If capnography is used and an ET tube is correctly placed in the trachea, a change in the waveform will be noted after exhalation.
- Watch for below normal values of end-tidal carbon dioxide in a digital read-out device.

Equipment

- BVM resuscitator
- End-tidal carbon dioxide detector
- ET or nasotracheal tube
- Oxygen

Preparation

- Examine all equipment, and check for defects.

- Wear appropriate PPE: goggles, face shield, gloves, and gown. Both the advanced and basic providers should wear appropriate PPE.

Procedure summary

You may be asked to retrieve the end-tidal carbon dioxide monitoring device to determine ET tube placement or to place the device yourself. You may also be requested to ventilate the patient while the advanced provider confirms tube placement.

End-tidal Carbon Dioxide Monitoring

BLS Provider Steps

1. Retrieve the carbon dioxide detector from the package.
2. Attach the detector to the ET or nasotracheal tube after it has been inserted into the trachea.
3. Ventilate the patient, if necessary.

PEDIATRIC BAG

A pediatric bag may be found in hospitals, ambulances, and other emergency vehicles. The pediatric bag contains resuscitation equipment that includes laryngoscope blades and handle, ET tubes, medications, and other equipment, all sized for the pediatric patient population. In addition, you may find a Broselow tape, which is used to measure the child from head to toe (Figure 6-4). The tape is color-coded; the color found at the child's feet after measuring from head to toe determines the size of equipment that may be used. Each

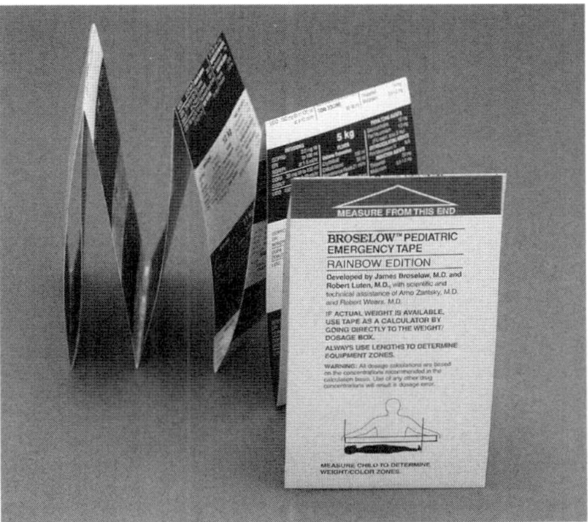

Figure 6-4 Pediatric Broselow (length-based) tape.

color on the Broselow tape contains information, such as the sizes of laryngoscope blades and ET tubes, as well as medications and doses. The equipment and medications can be found inside the pediatric bag in a small color-coded bag. The advanced provider may call out "the patient is a color blue," after measuring the patient with the Broselow tape. As the basic provider, you can retrieve the blue color bag found inside the pediatric bag and give it to the advanced provider.

Common Medical Emergencies

Objectives

After completing this chapter, you will be able to:
1. *Define the listed key terms.*
2. *Identify the signs and symptoms of various illnesses and injuries, and provide appropriate assistance to the advanced level provider.*

Key Terms

Asthma *Reversible airway disease in which the obstruction of air flow is caused by one or more of the following: spasm, secretions, and swelling—"the three Ss."*
Barrel chest *Large, rounded thorax.*
Chronic bronchitis *Form of chronic obstructive pulmonary disease that is characterized by recurrent excessive mucous secretion with obstruction of the smaller airways. The attacks may be accompanied by heart failure.*
Emphysema *Form of chronic obstructive pulmonary disease that is characterized by the destruction of the alveolar walls, leading to air trapping and enlarged alveoli. Emphysema commonly co-exists with chronic bronchitis and is virtually always found in the lungs of smokers.*
Hemoptysis *Coughing up blood from the lungs.*

Hypercholesterolemia *Higher-than-normal amounts of cholesterol in the blood.*

Infarction *Area of necrotic (dead) tissue as a result of the lack of blood flow to an area.*

Ischemia *Reduced or inadequate blood supply to the heart, thereby decreasing the oxygen supply to heart tissue (hypoxia).*

Parietal pleura *Serous membrane that lines the inside of the thoracic cavity.*

Pleural cavity *Potential space between the parietal and visceral pleurae.*

Pneumonia *Respiratory infection that may result from a bacterial, viral, or fungal organism.*

Pneumothorax *Air in the space between the parietal and visceral pleura (pleural cavity), causing the lungs to collapse. Pneumothorax causes atelectasis and can be spontaneous or related to trauma.*

Pulmonary edema *Accumulation of fluid in the alveoli and lung tissue.*

Pulmonary embolism *Free-flowing thrombus that lodges in a branch of the pulmonary artery, causing partial or total occlusion and sometimes infarction. The embolism may consist of clotted blood, fat, air, or amniotic fluid.*

Rhonchi *Abnormal lung sounds that indicate secretions are in the airway.*

Status asthmaticus *Severe, prolonged asthma attack that generally does not respond to normal treatments.*

Visceral pleura *Serous membrane on the outer surface of the lung.*

INTRODUCTION

If the patient does not have a patent airway, is unable to exchange gases appropriately, or is unable to circulate blood adequately, the outcome will be catastrophic. As a basic provider, your role is crucial in assisting in the management of the patient with respiratory and cardiac emergencies. Respiratory and cardiac disease may develop from a variety of origins; therefore a good understanding of the underlying pathologic conditions and a familiarity with potential treatments are important.

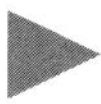 Remember, the ALS Passport generally consists of the five essential components that need to be carried out on all unstable or potentially unstable patients before or during transport to the hospital: (1) oxygen administration, (2) IV line, (3) pulse oximetry, (4) ECG application, and (5) glucose check (depending on your local protocols).

RESPIRATORY EMERGENCIES

DYSPNEA

Dyspnea, the sensation of breathlessness, is one of the most common complaints reported to emergency medical service (EMS) professionals. Familiarity with how to help treat the patient with dyspnea, as well as with the many different causes of dyspnea, is extremely important. Most causes are related to cardiopulmonary conditions such as congestive heart failure, chronic obstructive pulmonary disease, or trauma. You should always remember to ask the patient with dyspnea whether he or she is also experiencing chest pressure; you may find that the answer is often "yes."

CHRONIC OBSTRUCTIVE PULMONARY DISEASE

Chronic obstructive pulmonary disease (COPD) is a respiratory disease that is characterized by persistent obstruction to air flow. Emphysema, chronic bronchitis, and asthma are common conditions of COPD that can occur either alone or in conjunction with one another.

EMPHYSEMA

Emphysema is characterized by the destruction of the alveolar walls, which leads to air trapping and enlarged alveoli. Emphysema commonly co-exists with chronic bronchitis (Figure 7-1) and is virtually always found in the lungs of smokers.

Signs and symptoms

- Barrel chest
- Slender build
- Pursed lip breathing

Treatment

The patient with emphysema may complain of difficulty breathing and require 100% oxygen. In addition, the emphysemic patient may exhibit other complications. The prehospital care providers should never assume the patient with emphysema is concerned with only respiratory issues.

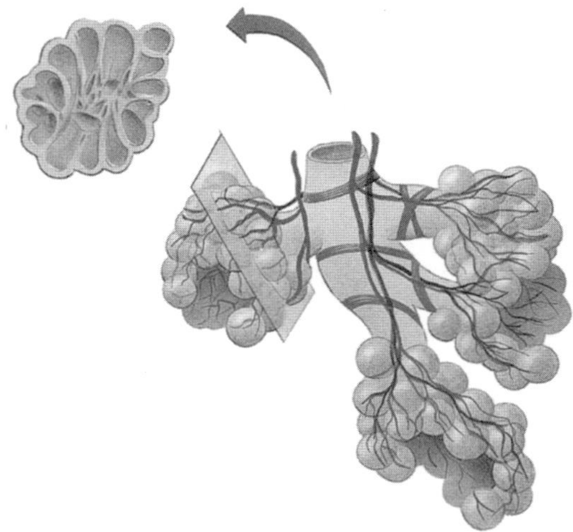

Figure 7-1 Emphysema.

> ### Emphysema
>
> #### Basic Life Support Provider Steps
>
> 1. Administer 100% oxygen via a nonrebreather mask at 15 L/min.
> 2. Place the patient in a position of comfort.
> 3. Prepare for a nebulizer treatment.
> 4. Take vital signs; complete an assessment.
> 5. Apply an ECG monitor.
> 6. Apply the pulse oximeter.
> 7. Check the glucose level.
> 8. Prepare for IV access.
> 9. Gather all the necessary equipment needed for endotracheal intubation; assist with intubation as necessary.

CHRONIC BRONCHITIS

Recurrent excessive mucous secretions with obstruction of the smaller airways characterize chronic bronchitis. It may be accompanied by heart failure (Figure 7-2).

Signs and symptoms

- Cyanosis
- Productive cough that worsens in the evening or with damp weather
- Fever, if the onset is acute
- Prolonged exhalation
- Rhonchi

Treatment

If the patient is in severe respiratory distress, administer 100% oxygen via a nonrebreather mask at 15 L/min. Monitor for respiratory depression. Intubation may be considered with severe respiratory distress. Two main causes of deterioration of the patient with chronic bronchitis are infection and heart failure.

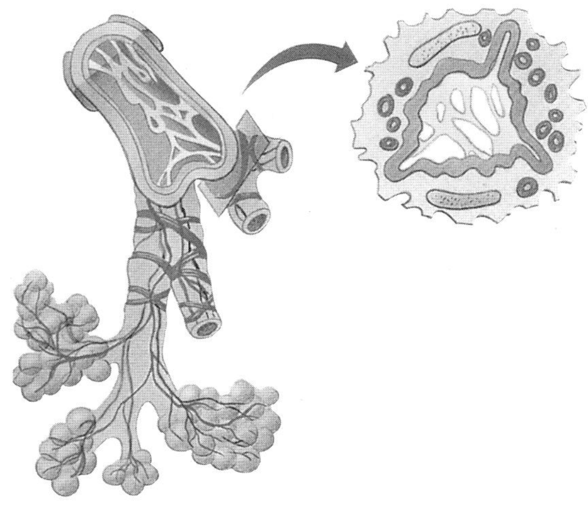

Figure 7-2 Chronic bronchitis.

Chronic Bronchitis

Basic Life Support Provider Steps

1. Administer 100% oxygen via a nonrebreather mask at 15 L/min.
2. Place the patient in a position of comfort.
3. Prepare for a nebulizer treatment.
4. Take vital signs; complete an assessment.
5. Apply an ECG monitor.
6. Apply a pulse oximeter.
7. Check glucose level.
8. Prepare for IV access.
9. Gather all the necessary equipment needed for endotracheal intubation; assist with intubation as necessary.

ASTHMA

Asthma is defined by dyspnea and wheezing as a result of generalized (reversible) narrowing of the smaller airways, which is usually caused by swelling, secretions, or spasm (or a combination thereof) (Figure 7-3).

Signs and symptoms

- Dyspnea
- Expiratory wheezing
- Chest tightness
- Cough
- Tachycardia
- Cyanosis
- Elevated blood pressure
- Patient is unable to speak a full sentence without taking a breath

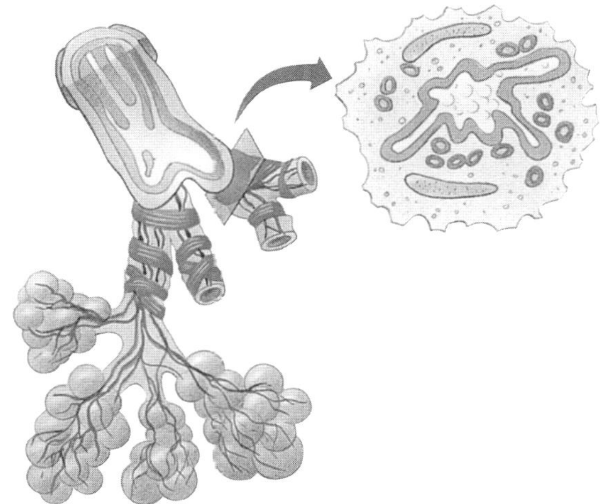

Figure 7-3   Asthma.

Treatment

The treatment of asthma is aimed at ensuring that the patient has an open airway, providing oxygen and trying to reverse bronchospasm. You may be directed to set up oxygen for the patient or to help deliver a bronchodilator such as Albuterol (or both). In severe cases, such as status asthmaticus, the patient may need to be intubated, and you may need to assist with intubation and other procedures. Remember, not every patient with asthma will exhibit wheezing, and it is important that you do not become completely focused on gadgets and forget to monitor the patient closely. Patients with asthma can deteriorate quickly.

Asthma

Basic Life Support Provider Steps

1. Ensure an open airway.
2. Apply 100% oxygen via a nonrebreather mask at 15 L/min.
3. Place the patient in a position of comfort.
4. Prepare for a nebulizer treatment.
5. Apply the ECG monitor.
6. Apply a pulse oximeter.
7. Check the glucose level.
8. Prepare for IV access.
9. Take vital signs; complete an assessment.
10. Assess breath sounds; note any wheezes, crackles, or rhonchi.
11. Perform a thorough head-to-toe assessment.
12. Gather the patient's medical history.
13. Assist with intubation, if necessary.

PULMONARY EMBOLISM

Pulmonary embolism is a free-flowing thrombus (clot) that lodges in a branch of the pulmonary artery, causing partial or total occlusion (blockage) and sometimes infarction (tissue death) (Figure 7-4). The embolus (foreign object) may consist of clotted blood, fat, air, or amniotic fluid. A thorough assessment of the patient who has the potential for a pulmonary embolism is important because determining a diagnosis may be difficult. A high index of suspicion should be maintained with the patient who has had recent surgery or prolonged immobilization, the woman on birth control, the patient with a recent trauma, and the individual with a history of atrial fibrillation. Pulmonary embolism is often confused with other conditions that cause chest pain, hypotension, or dyspnea.

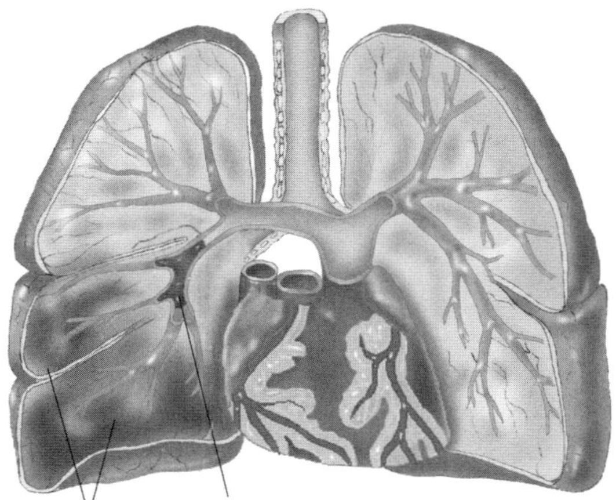

Figure 7-4 Pulmonary embolism.

Signs and symptoms

- Pleuritic chest pain that may be sudden
- Dyspnea
- Cyanosis
- Hemoptysis
- Diminished breath sounds over affected area
- Shock

Treatment

Early recognition is the key for treating an embolic emergency. You should maintain a high index of suspicion, especially with the following events: long-bone fracture, woman taking birth control, and patients who have had recent surgical procedures or prolonged periods of immobilization. Once in the emergency department, patients will receive IV heparin (a blood thinner) to prevent further pulmonary embolic events (portions of clotted blood that flows to and lodges in the pulmonary arterial blood vessels). Occasionally, fibrinolytic therapy is administered in the emergency department to lyse blood clots in the lung arteries just as it is given for myocardial infarction to lyse blood clots in the coronary arteries.

Pulmonary Embolism

Basic Life Support Provider Steps

1. Administer 100% oxygen via a nonrebreather mask at 15 L/min.
2. Take vital signs; complete an assessment .
3. Apply an ECG monitor.
4. Apply a pulse oximeter.
5. Check glucose level.
6. Prepare for IV access.
7. Monitor for signs and symptoms of shock.
8. Gather all the necessary equipment if endotracheal intubation is warranted; assist with intubation, if needed.
9. Transport as soon as possible.

PNEUMOTHORAX

A pneumothorax refers to air in the pleural cavity between the parietal and visceral pleura. This collection of air in the pleural cavity can cause the collapse of a lung and can be spontaneous or related to trauma (Figure 7-5).

Signs and symptoms

- Chest pain
- Dyspnea
- Cyanosis
- Diminished breath sounds over the affected lung field
- Tracheal deviation or mediastinal shift away from the affected side (tension pneumothorax)

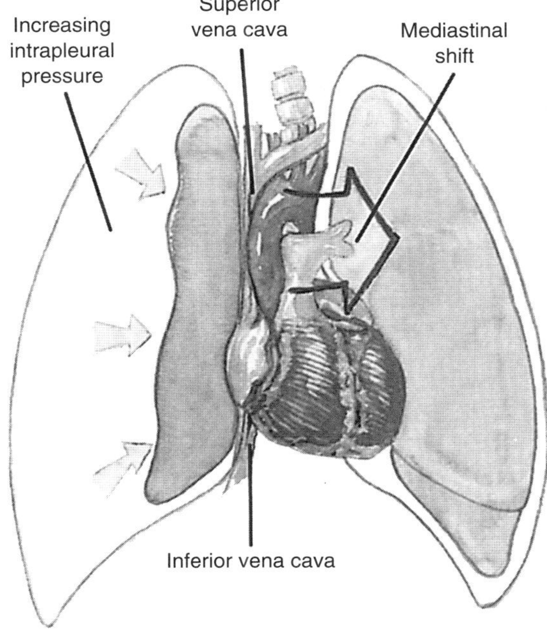

Figure 7-5 Pneumothorax.

- Jugular venous distention
- Shock
- Late signs, including tracheal deviation, jugular venous distention, and narrowing pulse pressure

Treatment

Chest decompression is used to expel air out of the pleural cavity during a tension pneumothorax. Once a tension pneumothorax has been determined, you should begin preparing the equipment that is needed for chest decompression. The advanced provider will be inserting a large-bore catheter into the affected side between the second and third intercostal region. Ensure that a 14 or 16 gauge IV catheter and iodine or alcohol are available to cleanse the site before insertion.

Pneumothorax

Basic Life Support Provider Steps

1. Administer 100% oxygen via a nonrebreather mask at 15 L/min.
2. Hold in-line cervical spine stabilization, if appropriate.
3. Assess bilateral breath sounds.
4. Take vital signs; complete an assessment.
5. Apply an ECG monitor.
6. Apply a pulse oximeter.
7. Check glucose level.
8. Prepare for IV access.
9. Monitor for signs and symptoms of shock.
10. Assist with chest decompression, if necessary.

PNEUMONIA

Pneumonia is a respiratory infection that may result from a bacterial, viral, or fungal organism (Figure 7-6).

Signs and symptoms

- Dyspnea
- Chills
- Fever
- Productive cough and purulent sputum
- Rhonchi
- Tachypnea
- Weakness and lethargy
- Wheezing

Treatment

Although treatment for pneumonia is best provided in the hospital, rapid assessment is a must for the patient with pneumonia. Pneumonia may be misdiagnosed as other respiratory conditions; therefore familiarity with the signs and symptoms may help more effectively treat the patient.

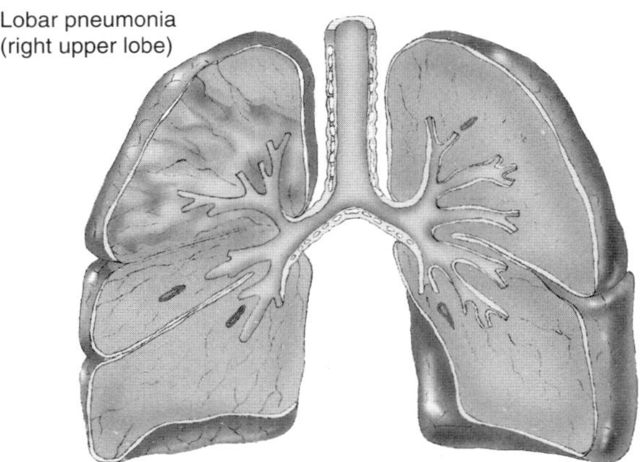

Figure 7-6 Pneumonia.

Pneumonia

Basic Life Support Provider Steps

1. Administer 100% oxygen via a nonrebreather mask at 15 L/min.
2. Assess bilateral breath sounds.
3. Place the patient in a position of comfort.
4. Prepare for a nebulizer treatment.
5. Take vital signs; complete an assessment.
6. Apply an ECG monitor.
7. Apply a pulse oximeter.
8. Check glucose level.
9. Prepare for IV access.
10. Gather all the necessary equipment if endotracheal intubation is warranted; assist with intubation, if needed.

CARDIAC EMERGENCIES

CONGESTIVE HEART FAILURE

When the heart fails to pump blood adequately, congestion occurs, which causes decreased cardiac output and increased systemic vascular resistance. Congestive heart failure may occur as a result of left- or right-sided heart failure. Left ventricular failure, for example, causes congestion in the heart and pulmonary edema, which causes a decrease in compliance, contractility, and elevated filling pressure (Figure 7-7).

Signs and symptoms

- Sudden dyspnea
- Pink frothy sputum
- Tachycardia

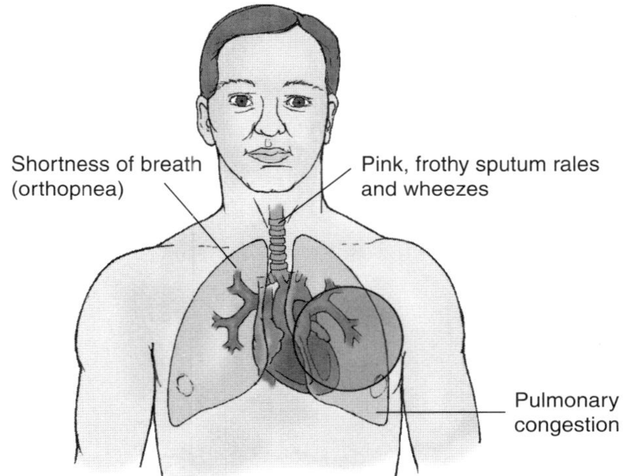

Figure 7-7 Congestive heart failure.

- Cool clammy skin
- Chest pain
- Rales or wheezing (usually an early sign)
- Patient usually reports using more pillows at night
- Increased dyspneic episodes throughout the day while working

Treatment

Congestive heart failure requires immediate treatment that consists of oxygen therapy, eliminating excess fluid, and alleviating other associated symptoms. The basic provider should become familiar with the pathophysiologic signs of congestive heart failure, along with the treatment modality that may be requested by the advanced provider.

Congestive Heart Failure

Basic Life Support Provider Steps

1. Administer 100% oxygen via a nonrebreather mask at 15 L/min.
2. Place the patient in a position of comfort.
3. Take vital signs; complete an assessment.
4. Apply an ECG monitor.
5. Apply a pulse oximeter.
6. Check glucose level.
7. Prepare for IV access.
8. Assist with the administration of sublingual nitroglycerin.
9. Retrieve Lasix; assist with preparation of the medication.
10. Retrieve morphine sulfate; assist with preparation of the medication.
11. Prepare for endotracheal intubation, if warranted; assist with intubation, if needed.

CORONARY HEART DISEASE

Coronary heart disease is caused by a disruption in the flow of oxygen and nutrients to the heart muscle. This disruption results in damage to the heart muscle and can potentially lead to death.

To function properly, the heart muscle needs a constant supply of blood to carry adequate levels of oxygen and nutrients. The coronary arteries are the key blood vessels responsible for feeding oxygenated blood to the heart. Any disruption in the flow of blood through the coronary arteries can lead to an inadequate supply of oxygen and, over time, lead to death of the affected portion of the heart muscle (infarction).

Coronary artery disease (CAD) is one of the most common causes of disruption. CAD may be the result of high cholesterol, smoking, obesity, diabetes, older age, or hypertension, among other factors. The result of CAD is a buildup of plaque in the coronary arteries. This buildup reduces the flow of blood to the heart, which can then lead to myocardial infarction.

You should remember that with any cardiac emergency, "time is muscle." The quicker the prehospital team intervenes and the patient is transported to the hospital while providing appropriate field management, the better the chance for survival. Reviewing all the different types of cardiac emergencies is beyond the scope of this text. Nevertheless, some of the most common emergent complaints are discussed to help you assist the ALS team.

ANGINA PECTORIS

Angina pectoris is chest pain or discomfort that occurs as a result of inadequate amounts of oxygen reaching the heart.

Types of angina

STABLE ANGINA. This type of angina is predictable in nature. For example, chest pain may occur with certain activities such as exercising. Running, lifting, or any activity that makes the heart's demand for oxygen exceed the oxygen supply are examples of stable angina. Usually the chest pain lasts less than 5 minutes and can be reversed by stopping the stressful activity or with treatments such as oxygen administration and nitroglycerin.

UNSTABLE ANGINA. This type of angina is less predictable. The chest pain can occur while the individual is at rest, and the episodes can occur more frequently and last longer than stable angina. Unstable angina usually precedes acute myocardial infarction.

Signs and symptoms

- Dyspnea
- Diaphoresis

- Nausea
- Vomiting
- Heartburn
- Indigestion
- Palpitations (sensation in the chest that "feels like my heart is racing")
- Dizziness
- Description of tightness or constriction around the heart or in the chest area
- Pain that may travel down one or both arms, in the jaw, or in the back

Treatment

Although angina pectoris is a transient event, it should not be considered a mild occurrence, especially when the patient tells you that his or her chest discomfort is no longer predictable; that is, it no longer occurs only during physical exertion, for example. The treatment of choice for angina pectoris is sublingual nitroglycerin and aspirin but only after a blood pressure check.

Angina Pectoris

Basic Life Support Provider Steps

1. Administer 100% oxygen via a nonrebreather mask at 15 L/min.
2. Take vital signs; complete an assessment.
3. Apply an ECG monitor.
4. Apply a pulse oximeter.
5. Check glucose level.
6. Assist with administration of sublingual nitroglycerin.
7. Prepare for IV access.

MYOCARDIAL INFARCTION

Myocardial infarction or heart attack is the primary medical emergency of the cardiovascular system. Although myocardial infarction may strike suddenly and many times without warning, the cause is a slow and progressive deterioration of the heart's major pathways for blood supply through the coronary arteries. Causes of narrowing in the coronary artery include atherosclerosis, embolus, and coronary spasm (Figure 7-8).

Signs and symptoms

- Chest pain, back pain, toothache, left or right arm pain
- Pain described as constricting, pressure (may or may not be relieved by positioning or nitroglycerin)
- Dyspnea
- Diaphoresis
- Nausea
- Vomiting
- Ashen or pale skin
- Irregular pulse
- Diabetes (may be pain free and may have other complaints that mask the more common signs and symptoms of myocardial infarction)
- Most patients die within $2\frac{1}{2}$ hours from the onset of the pain, depending on the injury or infarct progression

Treatment

Remember, "Time is muscle." As a basic provider, you need to be familiar with the equipment and some of the treatment regimens before the emergency occurs to help reduce on-the-scene time. The quicker the prehospital intervention occurs, the better the chance of myocardial muscle survivability. In addition, the key term *MONA* stands for morphine sulfate, oxygen, nitroglycerin, and aspirin. The advanced provider turns to this treatment regimen when treating an acute myocardial infarction in the prehospital setting.

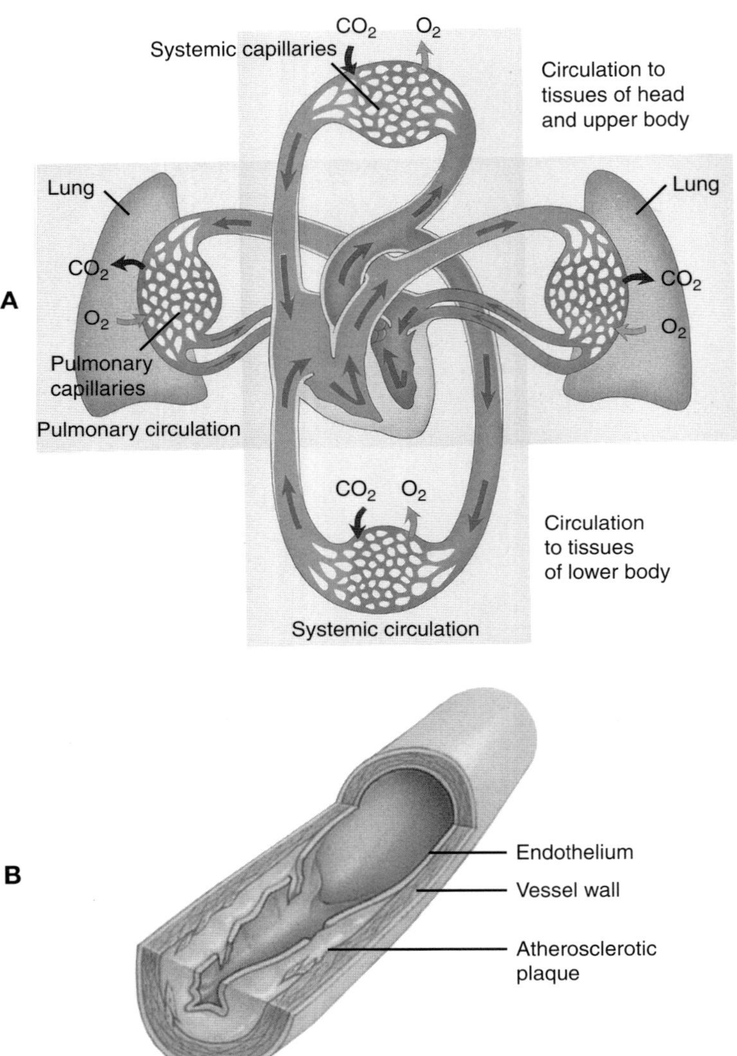

Figure 7-8 **A,** Normal blood flow. **B,** Atherosclerosis.

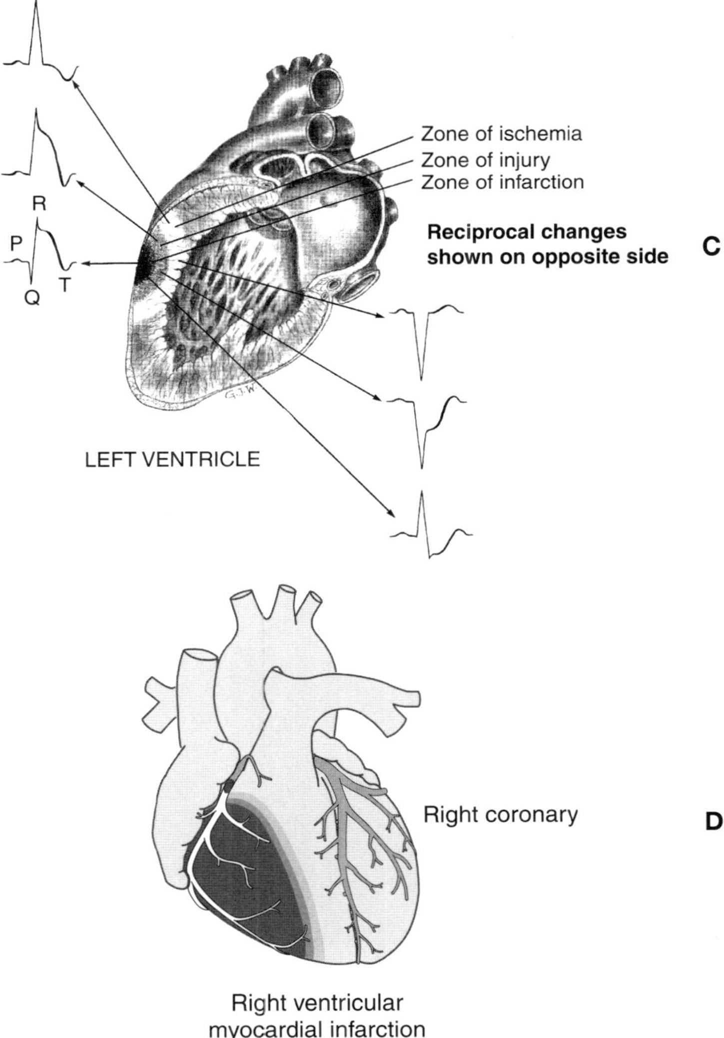

Figure 7-8—cont'd **C,** Ischemia. **D,** Myocardial infarction.

Myocardial Infarction

Basic Life Support Provider Steps

1. Administer 100% oxygen via a nonrebreather mask at 15 L/min.
2. Take vital signs; complete an assessment.
3. Apply an ECG monitor.
4. Apply a pulse oximeter.
5. Gather baby aspirin; ensure aspirin is available for the advanced provider.
6. Gather sublingual nitroglycerin; double check with the advanced provider before administering.
7. Prepare for IV access.
8. Draw blood.
9. Complete a thrombolytic inclusion and exclusion criteria sheet.

Putting It All Together

Now it is time to put this information all together. The following scenarios are written to help you apply this new knowledge when assisting an advanced provider. In the space provided after each scenario you will be asked to describe the course of action needed from the basic provider's point of view. Through practice and having a planned approach, you can function as an integral part of the ALS team.

Remember, when assisting the advanced provider, the following five essential steps must be accomplished before or during transport to the hospital for all patients who require ALS:

1. Oxygen administration
2. IV line
3. Pulse oximetry
4. ECG application
5. Glucose check (depending on local protocols)

CASE STUDY 1

You are dispatched to a 47-year-old man who is complaining of chest pressure. On arrival, you find the man sitting on a bus bench. He tells the crew that he is experiencing a lot of pressure in his chest. As the advanced provider interviews the patient, what can you do as the basic provider?

CASE STUDY 2

You are dispatched to a man who is in cardiac arrest. On arrival, you notice the man lying supine in his front yard. During the initial assessment, it is noted that the man is pulseless and apneic. No trauma is noted on the patient. How do you assist the advanced provider?

CASE STUDY 3

You are dispatched to a 72-year-old woman who is complaining of shortness of breath. On arrival, you find the patient sitting up in bed and in severe distress. She is cool, diaphoretic, and anxious. Lung sounds reveal crackles (rales) and wheezing throughout all lung fields. The advanced provider alerts the team that the patient may have congestive heart failure. Vital signs are blood pressure 180/110, heart rate 110, and respiratory rate 28. How do you assist the advanced provider?

CASE STUDY 4

You are dispatched to a man who has fallen at a local supermarket. On arrival, you find the 67-year-old man sitting up in severe respiratory distress. The patient can barely speak. However, he manages to say that he has a history of asthma and does not have his inhaler with him. Breath sounds reveal inspiratory and expiratory wheezing throughout all lung fields. The patient's vital signs are blood pressure 162/88, heart rate 110, and respiratory rate 32; his skin is cool and diaphoretic. The advanced provider informs you that the patient is experiencing an acute asthma attack. How do you assist the advanced provider?

CASE STUDY 5

You are dispatched to an unresponsive man at a local bar. On arrival, you find the patient in a car responding only to painful stimuli. No trauma to the patient is noted. The patient's breath sounds are clear, and his skin is cool, pale, and diaphoretic. His vital signs are blood pressure 150/72, heart rate 96, and respiratory rate 24. The advanced provider informs you that this individual will be treated as an unresponsive patient. How do you assist the advanced provider?

CASE STUDY 6

You are dispatched to an 18-year-old woman who is complaining of an acute onset of shortness of breath and chest pain. In addition, the patient related that she was watching television when she began experiencing chest pain and shortness of breath. The patient denies any medical history, but she is taking birth control pills. In addition, she states that she smokes one pack of cigarettes per day. The advanced provider auscultates breath sounds and notices localized wheezing on the right side. How would you assist the advanced provider?

Case Study 7

You are dispatched to a near drowning accident. On arrival, you find a 2-year-old child at the side of a pool; cardiopulmonary resuscitation (CPR) is in progress. How would you assist the advanced provider?

Case Study 8

You respond to a local park where you find a 36-year-old woman who is complaining of a shortness of breath. The advanced provider auscultates breath sounds, and expiratory wheezing is noted bilaterally. In addition, the patient relates that she feels itchy all over. You notice urticaria on the patient's chest and extremities. How would you assist the advanced provider?

CASE STUDY 9

You respond to a man who has fallen from a ladder. The patient is found unconscious, unresponsive, and not breathing. The patient has a laceration on the frontal region over his left eye. The patient's blood pressure is 180/110, and his heart rate is 62. How can you assist the advanced provider?

Case Study 10

You respond to a nursing facility where an 86-year-old woman is found lying in bed unconscious and unresponsive. The patient's blood pressure is 110/78, heart rate 72, and respiratory rate 26. The advanced provider checks the glucose and relates to you a reading of 36 mg/dL. How can you assist the advanced provider?

Answers to Case Studies from Chapter 8

CASE STUDY 1

- Administer 100% oxygen via a nonrebreather mask at 15 L/min.
- Record vital signs, complete physical examination, and take SAMPLE survey.
- Apply an ECG monitor.
- Set up pulse oximetry.
- Check glucose level.
- Assist with the following:
  - ► Administer baby aspirin.
  - ► Administer sublingual nitroglycerin.
  - ► Administer IV NS, preferably with a double lumen catheter.
  - ► Blood draw.
- Complete a thrombolytic inclusion-exclusion criteria sheet.
- Administer morphine sulfate, if indicated.

CASE STUDY 2

- Complete an initial assessment.
- Conduct CPR.
- Apply ECG monitor in case defibrillation is immediately warranted.

- Establish airway, and administer 100% oxygen via BVM.
- Assist with the administration of the following:
  - Establish endotracheal intubation.
  - Establish an IV line.
  - ALS medication.
  - Check glucose level.

Case Study 3

- Administer 100% oxygen via a nonrebreather mask at 15 L/min.
- Sit the patient in a position of comfort.
- Record vital signs, and complete a physical examination.
- Set up pulse oximetry.
- Apply an ECG monitor.
- Assist with the administration of the following:
  - Check glucose level (90 to 120 mg/dL is a good range).
  - Establish an IV NS (watch out for overloading the patient).
  - Administer nitroglycerin.
  - Administer furosemide (Lasix).
  - Begin nebulizer treatment if wheezing is heard on auscultation.
  - Administer morphine sulfate.
  - Establish ET intubation.

Case Study 4

- Administer 100% oxygen via a nonrebreather mask at 15 L/min.
- Sit the patient in a position of comfort.
- Record vital signs, and complete physical examination.

- Apply an ECG monitor.
- Set up pulse oximetry.
- Assist with the administration of the following:
  - Check glucose level.
  - Establish IV access.
  - Begin nebulizer treatment.

Case Study 5

- Administer 100% oxygen via a nonrebreather mask at 15 L/min.
- Maintain patient's airway.
- Record vital signs, and complete a physical examination.
- Apply an ECG monitor.
- Set up pulse oximetry.
- Check glucose level.
- Establish IV access.
- Administer naloxone (Narcan).
- Administer 50% dextrose.

Case Study 6

- Administer 100% oxygen via a nonrebreather mask at 15 L/min.
- Place the patient in position of comfort.
- Record vital signs, and complete a physical examination.
- Apply an ECG monitor.
- Set up pulse oximetry.
- Check glucose level.
- Assist with the administration of the following:
  - Establish IV access.
  - Begin nebulizer treatment.

Case Study 7

- Complete initial assessment.
- Begin CPR.
- Apply an ECG monitor in case defibrillation is immediately warranted.
- Establish an open airway, and administer 100% oxygen via BVM through oral airway.
- Maintain cervical spine stabilization.
- Make available a pediatric bag and Broselow tape.
- Set up ET intubation (make available one large tube and one small tube).
- Assist with the administration of the following:
  - ▸ Establish an IV line (IO).
  - ▸ Administer ALS medication.
  - ▸ Check glucose level.
  - ▸ Warm patient.

Case Study 8

- Administer 100% oxygen via a nonrebreather mask at 15 L/min.
- Place the patient in position of comfort.
- Record vital signs, and complete a physical examination.
- Apply an ECG monitor.
- Set up pulse oximetry.
- Check glucose level.
- Assist with the administration of the following:
  - ▸ Establish IV access.
  - ▸ Begin nebulizer treatment.
  - ▸ Administer epinephrine.
  - ▸ Administer diphenhydramine (Benadryl).

CASE STUDY 9

- Maintain an open airway.
- Administer 100% oxygen via a BVM with an oral airway at 15 L/min.
- Provide manual stabilization of the cervical spine.
- Assist with the administration of the following:
  - ▸ Establish ET and bag-valve ventilation.
  - ▸ Record vital signs, complete a physical examination, and take a SAMPLE survey.
- Apply an ECG monitor.
- Set up pulse oximetry.
- Check glucose level.
- Assist with the administration of the following:
  - ▸ Administer IV NS.
  - ▸ Dress the wound.

CASE STUDY 10

- Administer 100% oxygen via a nonrebreather mask at 15 L/min.
- Record vital signs, and complete a physical examination.
- Apply an ECG monitor.
- Set up pulse oximetry.
- Assist with the administration of the following:
  - ▸ Check glucose level.
  - ▸ Establish IV access.
  - ▸ Administer 50% dextrose.

Acetylcholine Type of neurotransmitter that stimulates the parasympathetic nervous system.

Acidosis Abnormal increase of hydrogen ions (acid) in the blood.

Acute respiratory distress syndrome Insufficiency of the respiratory system that is the result of damage to the lungs. Causes leakage of fluid into the alveoli.

Adrenergic Pertains to sympathetic nerve fibers or epinephrine-like substances as neurotransmitters.

Air embolism Abnormal presence of air in the cardiovascular system. When air is introduced into the vein, an embolism may result, which can obstruct blood flow.

Alveolus Tiny air sacs located at the most distal end of the air passages.

Anemia Decreased hemoglobin level in the blood.

Antidysrhythmic agent Medication used to suppress cardiac dysrhythmias.

Aortic semilunar valve Determines the outflow of blood from the ventricles. It is located at the exit point of the left ventricle, where it opens into the aorta.

Apex of the heart Lower cone-shaped portion of the heart.

Apex of the lung Upper portion of the lung.

Ascites Abnormal pooling of fluid in the abdominal cavity, which contains large amounts of protein and other cells.

Aseptic Procedures used to reduce the number of microorganisms and to prevent their spread.

Asthma Reversible airway disease in which the obstruction of air flow is caused by one or more of the following: spasm, secretions, and swelling—"the three Ss."

Atelectasis Complete or partial collapse of the alveoli in certain sections of the lungs because of pressure or under use.

Atria Upper chambers of the heart.

Atrioventricular node Specialized cells located in the lower portion of the right atrium that allows electrical impulses from the sinoatrial node to travel into the ventricles.

Atrioventricular valves Heart valves located between the atria and ventricles.

Autonomic nervous system Part of the nervous system that regulates involuntary vital functions such as glandular, cardiac, and smooth muscle activity.

Baroreceptor Detects a change in blood pressure. Baroreceptors are located in the carotid arteries and in the aorta.

Barrel chest Large, rounded thorax.

Base of the heart Top part of the heart located near the second intercostal space.

Base of the lung Bottom portion of the lung.

Bicuspid or *mitral valve* Valve located between the left atrium and left ventricle.

Bronchioles Small tubes that branch off the left or right bronchus and lead to the alveolar sacs.

Bronchoconstrictor Substance that causes constriction (narrowing) of the bronchial smooth muscle-restricting airflow.

Bronchodilator Substance that causes relaxation (widening) of the bronchial smooth muscle, thereby improving airflow.

Bronchus Large airway located in the lungs that connects the trachea with the bronchioles.

Bundle branches Branches of specialized electrical conducting cells that extend from the bundle of His into the ventricles, dividing into three branches.

Bundle of His Cardiac fibers that connect the atrioventricular node and the two bundle branches.

Butterfly needle Used for cannulating small veins, the butterfly needle has a winged appearance.

Carina Point at which the trachea divides into the right and left bronchi.

Catecholamine Any group of sympathomimetic agents.

Catheter shear Teflon catheter that is introduced over the needle that may be inclined to shear once the catheter is advanced and then pulled back.

Chemoreceptors Sensory nerve cells located in the carotid arteries and aortic arch that detect changes in oxygen, carbon dioxide, and pH levels.

Chemstrip reading Similar to a glucometer reading (except when the blood is wiped off after 60 seconds), a chemstrip reading is compared with a color-coded system on the side of the bottle in which it is stored. Under the matching color system, a numerical reading indicates the amount of glucose.

Chronic bronchitis Form of chronic obstructive pulmonary disease that is characterized by recurrent excessive mucous secretion with obstruction of the smaller airways. The attacks may be accompanied by heart failure.

Chronotrope Substance that affects the heart rate. A positive chronotrope increases heart rate, whereas a negative chronotrope decreases it.

Coronary arteries Responsible for supplying the heart with oxygen and nutrients. The left coronary artery is typically referred to as the "widow maker" because severe occlusion of this vessel prevents blood flow to both the left anterior descending and the left circumflex artery (branches of the left coronary artery). Death would be imminent.

Cricoid cartilage Ring-shaped cartilage in the larynx.

Cricoid pressure Pressure applied over the cricoid cartilage to reduce the possibility of regurgitation and therefore aspiration by occluding the esophagus during airway maneuvers. This procedure may also be referred to as Sellick's maneuver and is critically important when managing the airway of a patient who has already increased gastric distention as a result of BVM ventilation.

Defibrillation The discharge of electricity from a medical device into the chest when the heart has unstable or dysfunctional electrical activity.

Diaphoresis Excessive sweating.

Diuresis Increases urine secretion.

Dyspnea Uncomfortable sensation of breathlessness.

Dysrhythmia Any cardiac rhythm other than a normal sinus rhythm.

Emphysema Form of chronic obstructive pulmonary disease that is characterized by the destruction of the alveolar walls, leading to air trapping and enlarged alveoli. Emphysema commonly co-exists with chronic bronchitis and is virtually always found in the lungs of smokers.

Endocardium Innermost layer of the heart.

Endotracheal tube Plastic tube that is placed in the trachea to provide an airway.

End-tidal carbon dioxide capnometry Sensor device attached to an endotracheal (ET) tube, which detects and measures the presence of and changes in carbon dioxide in exhaled air on a continuous basis.

End-tidal carbon dioxide detector Sensor device attached to an ET tube that detects the presence of carbon dioxide in exhaled air.

Epicardium Thin, outermost layer of the heart.

Epigastrium Upper region of the stomach.

External cardiac pacing Electrical pacing with a medical device that replaces or overrides existing dysfunctional cardiac electrical activity.

Fluid overload Excessive fluid accumulation in the body, which causes problems with circulation.

Foci Specific locations; that is, locations where electrical activity occur in the heart.

Gag reflex Response to stimulation of the upper palate or posterior oropharynx, causing many individuals to gag or vomit or both.

Glucometer Small machine that calculates and displays the patient's glucose reading.

Gtts Abbreviation for drops.

Hemodynamically unstable Unstable vital signs.

Hemoptysis Coughing up blood from the lungs.

Histamine blocker Chemical that blocks histamine receptors, thus preventing the release of histamine.

Hypercholesterolemia Higher-than-normal amounts of cholesterol in the blood.

Hypoxic drive Respiration stimulated by the amount of oxygen in the blood.

Infarction Area of necrotic (dead) tissue as a result of the lack of blood flow to an area.

Infection Invasion of the body by germs that reproduce and multiply, causing disease by local cell injury, release of poisons, or germ antibody reaction in the cells. Infection may result at the IV site if poor aseptic technique is used.

Infiltration Fluid passing into tissues. Infiltration can result from IV cannulation.

Inotrope Substance that improves the contractility of a muscle, particularly the heart.

Ischemia Reduced or inadequate blood supply to the heart, thereby decreasing the oxygen supply to the heart tissue (hypoxia).

KVO Abbreviation for *keep vein open.*

Lancet Short, pointed blade used to obtain a drop of blood.

Laryngoscope Instrument that consists of a handle and blade. It is used for examining the larynx and for assisting in the completion of procedures related to airway and pulmonary maintenance, such as foreign body removal and ET intubation.

Larynx (voice box) Organ in the neck that consists of the thyroid cartilage, cricoid cartilage, and vocal cords. The larynx has three important functions: (1) control of airflow during breathing, (2) protection of the airway, and (3) production of sound for speech.

Lead Electrical connection attached to the body for the purpose of monitoring physiologic electrical activity.

Lower airway Structures located below the larynx in which gas exchange occurs.

Macrodrip IV set Device used to deliver large amounts of IV solution.

Magill forceps Elongated pair of forceps used to advance an ET tube during intubation or to remove a foreign body during complete airway obstruction.

Mediastinum Area between the lungs that includes the heart, esophagus, and great vessels.

Microdrip IV set Device used to deliver small amounts of IV solution.

Minute ventilation Total amount of air breathed in and out in 1 minute. Calculated by multiplying the lung tidal volume by the respiratory rate.

Myocardium Thick middle layer of the heart.

Nasotracheal intubation Procedure involving the placement of an ET tube into the trachea through the nose.

Orotracheal intubation Procedure involving the placement of an ET tube into the trachea through the oral cavity.

P wave Represents atrial depolarization.

Parasympathetic nervous system Subdivision of the autonomic nervous system that is involved in activating vegetative functions such as urination, defecation, and digestion.

Parasympatholytic substance Blocks the action of the parasympathetic nervous system.

Parasympathomimetic substance Has effects that resemble those of the parasympathetic system.

Parietal pleura Serous membrane that lines the inside of the thoracic cavity.

Pericardium Thick, protective sac that surrounds the heart.

Pleural cavity Potential space between the parietal and visceral pleurae.

Pneumonia Respiratory infection that may result from a bacterial, viral, or fungal organism.

Pneumothorax Air in the space between the parietal and visceral pleura (pleural cavity), causing the lungs to collapse. Pneumothorax causes atelectasis and can be spontaneous or related to trauma.

PR interval Represents the length of time required for the atria to depolarize and the delay of the impulse through the atrioventricular (AV) junction. Normally, the PR interval measures 0.12 to 0.20 seconds.

Pulmonary edema Accumulation of fluid in the alveoli and lung tissue.

Pulmonary embolism Free-flowing thrombus that lodges in a branch of the pulmonary artery, causing partial or total occlusion and sometimes infarction. The embolism may consist of clotted blood, fat, air, or amniotic fluid.

Pulmonary semilunar valve Determines the outflow of blood from the ventricles. It is located at the exit point of the right ventricle, where it opens into the pulmonary arteries.

Pulse oximeter Device that indirectly measures the saturation of oxygen in the hemoglobin contained in red blood cells.

Purkinje fibers Elaborate web of specialized electrically conducting fibers that extend through the bundle of His and bundle branches throughout the myocardial tissue for the purpose of propagating electrical impulses to the muscle to cause contractions.

Pyrogenic reactions Reaction that may cause shock, fever, headache, or backache.

QRS complex Represents ventricular depolarization.
- Q wave is the first negative, downward deflection, deflection after the P wave.
- R wave is the first positive, upward deflection, after the P wave.
- QRS complex usually measure between 0.04 to 0.12 seconds.
- S wave is the negative deflection after the R wave.

QT interval Represents total ventricular activity. QT interval is the total time required for ventricular depolarization and repolarization to take place.

Respiratory rate Number of breaths per minute (bpm).

Rhonchi Abnormal lung sounds that indicate secretions are in the airway.

Sellick's maneuver *See* Cricoid pressure.

Sinoatrial node Normal pacemaker of the heart that typically fires at a rate between 60 and 100 bpm in adults.

ST segment Represents early repolarization of the right and left ventricles. The ST segment begins with the end of the QRS complex and ends with the onset of the T wave. When elevated or depressed, it generally represents injury to the myocardium (heart muscle) as a result of decreased blood flow through the coronary (heart) arteries.

Status asthmaticus Severe, prolonged asthma attack that generally does not respond to normal treatments.

Status epilepticus Recurrent generalized seizure during which no resumption of consciousness occurs; a seizure that lasts longer than 15 minutes.

Stylet Metal probe or rod that passes through a catheter, needle, or tube. This device is used to stiffen an otherwise flexible tool to facilitate insertion. A stylet is inserted to form the ET tube and is removed after orotracheal intubation.

Surfactant Lipoprotein secreted by the alveolar cells, which reduces the surface tension in the alveoli, allowing the alveolar sacs to stay open to permit gas exchange.

Sympathetic nervous system Subdivision of the autonomic nervous system that is involved in preparing the body for physical activity.

Sympatholytic substance Blocks the action of the sympathetic nervous system.

Sympathomimetic substance Mimics or stimulates the sympathetic nervous system.

Synchronized cardioversion Discharge of electricity from a medical device into the chest. It is synchronized with ventricular depolarization to convert an unstable rapid cardiac rhythm to a stable normal (sinus) heart rhythm.

Syncope Fainting episode.

T wave Represents ventricular repolarization.

Thrombophlebitis Inflammation of the vein accompanied by a clot. Prolonged IV therapy can cause thrombophlebitis.

Tidal volume Amount of air breathed in and out with each breath (approximately 500 mL for an adult).

TKO Abbreviation for *to keep open.*

Transcutaneous cardiac pacing *See* External cardiac pacing.

Tricuspid valve Valve between the right atrium and right ventricle.

Upper airway Airway structures above the larynx.

Urticaria Skin reaction that is characterized by a rash and accompanied by itching.

Vasopressor Substance that causes vasoconstriction.

Ventricles Lower chambers of the heart.

Visceral pleura Serous membrane on the outer surface of the lung.

Vocal cords Most important part of the larynx made of muscle and cartilage. It is covered with a thick layer of mucosa, which is critical for the production of sound for speech and for appropriately opening and closing the airway for breathing and swallowing.

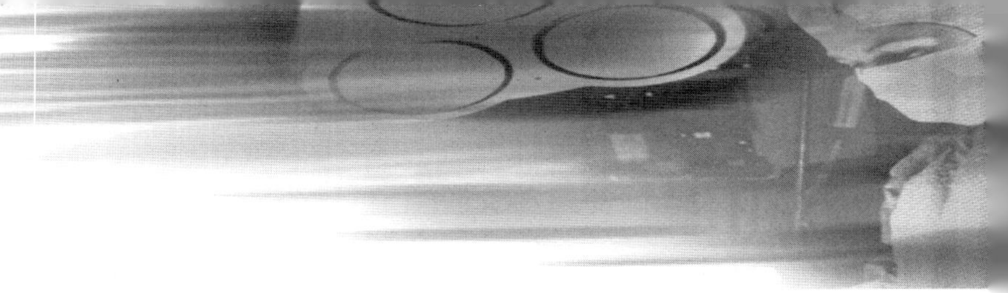

SUGGESTED READINGS

Aehlert B: *ACLS quick review study guide*, ed 2, St Louis, 2002, Mosby.

Aehlert B: *ECGs made easy*, ed 2, St Louis, 2002, Mosby.

Anderson KN, Anderson LE, Glanze WD, editors: *Mosby's medical, nursing, & allied health dictionary*, ed 6, St Louis, 2002, Mosby.

Gould B: *Pathophysiology for the health professions*, ed 2, Philadelphia, 2002, WB Saunders.

Herlihy B, Maebius N: *The human body in health and illness*, ed 2, Philadelphia, 2000, WB Saunders.

Huszar R: *Basic dysrhythmias interpretation and management*, ed 3, St Louis, 2002, Mosby.

McSwain N, Paturas J: *The basic EMT comprehensive prehospital patient care*, ed 2, St Louis, 2003, Mosby.

NAEMT: *PHTLS basic and advanced prehospital trauma life support*, ed 5, St Louis, 2003, Mosby.

Sanders M: *Mosby's paramedic textbook*, ed 2, St Louis, 2001, Mosby.

Shade B et al: *Mosby's EMT-intermediate textbook*, ed 2, St Louis, 2002, Mosby.

Thelan L et al: *Critical care nursing: diagnosis and management*, ed 2, St Louis, 1998, Mosby.

Thibodeau G, Patton K: *Anthony's textbook of anatomy & physiology*, ed 16, St Louis, 1999, Mosby.

Wilson SF: *Respiratory disorders*, St Louis, 1990, Mosby.

ILLUSTRATION CREDITS

Figure 1-1 (page 3): McSwain N, Paturas J: *The basic EMT: comprehensive prehospital patient care*, ed 2, St Louis, 2003, Mosby.

Figure 1-2 (page 5): Herlihy B, Maebius N: *The human body in health and illness*, ed 2, Philadelphia, 2000, WB Saunders.

Figure 2-1 (page 11): Sanders M: *Mosby's paramedic textbook revised*, ed 2, St Louis, 2001, Mosby.

Figure 2-2 (page 12): Cairo J: *Mosby's respiratory care equipment*, ed 6, St Louis, 1999, Mosby.

Figure 2-3 (page 13): Sanders M: *Mosby's paramedic textbook revised*, ed 2, St Louis, 2001, Mosby.

Figure 2-4 (page 13): Sanders M: *Mosby's paramedic textbook revised*, ed 2, St Louis, 2001, Mosby.

Figure 2-5 (page 14): Sanders M: *Mosby's paramedic textbook revised,* ed 2, St Louis, 2001, Mosby.

Figure 2-6 (page 14): Sanders M: *Mosby's paramedic textbook revised,* ed 2, St Louis, 2001, Mosby.

Figure 2-7 (page 15): Sanders M: *Mosby's paramedic textbook revised,* ed 2, St Louis, 2001, Mosby.

Figure 2-8 (page 20): NAEMT: *Prehospital trauma life support,* ed 5, St Louis, 2003, Mosby.

Figure 2-9 (page 25): Shade B et al: *Mosby's EMT-intermediate textbook,* ed 2, St Louis, 2002, Mosby.

Figure 2-10 (page 29): Sanders M: *Mosby's paramedic textbook revised,* ed 2, St Louis, 2001, Mosby.

Figure 2-11 (page 30): NAEMT: *Prehospital trauma life support,* ed 5, St Louis, 2003, Mosby.

Figure 3-1 (page 37): Aehlert B: *ECGs made easy,* ed 2, St Louis, 2002, Mosby.

Figure 3-2 (page 41): Huszar R: *Basic dysrhythmias interpretation and management,* ed 3, St Louis, 2002, Mosby.

Figure 3-3 (page 44): Aehlert B: *ECGs made easy,* ed 2, St Louis, 2002, Mosby.

Figure 3-4 (page 50): Sanders M: *Mosby's paramedic textbook revised,* ed 2, St Louis, 2001, Mosby.

Figure 3-5 (page 51): Sanders M: *Mosby's paramedic textbook revised,* ed 2, St Louis, 2001, Mosby.

Figure 3-6 (page 52): Sanders M: *Mosby's paramedic textbook revised,* ed 2, St Louis, 2001, Mosby.

Figure 3-7 (page 53): Aehlert B: *ECGs made easy,* ed 2, St Louis, 2002, Mosby.

Figure 3-8 (page 54): Aehlert B: *ECGs made easy,* ed 2, St Louis, 2002, Mosby.

Figure 3-9 (page 55): Sanders M: *Mosby's paramedic textbook revised,* ed 2, St Louis, 2001, Mosby.

Figure 3-10 (page 56): Aehlert B: *ECGs made easy,* ed 2, St Louis, 2002, Mosby.

Figure 3-11 (page 57): Sanders M: *Mosby's paramedic textbook revised,* ed 2, St Louis, 2001, Mosby.

Figure 3-12 (page 58): Sanders M: *Mosby's paramedic textbook revised,* ed 2, St Louis, 2001, Mosby.

Figure 3-13 (page 59): Aehlert B: *ECGs made easy,* ed 2, St Louis, 2002, Mosby.

Figure 3-14 (page 60): Sanders M: *Mosby's paramedic textbook revised,* ed 2, St Louis, 2001, Mosby.

Figure 3-15 (page 61): Sanders M: *Mosby's paramedic textbook revised,* ed 2, St Louis, 2001, Mosby.

Figure 3-16 (page 62): Aehlert B: *ECGs made easy,* ed 2, St Louis, 2002, Mosby.

Figure 3-17 (page 63): Aehlert B: *ECGs made easy,* ed 2, St Louis, 2002, Mosby.

Figure 3-18 (page 64): Sanders M: *Mosby's paramedic textbook revised,* ed 2, St Louis, 2001, Mosby.

Figure 3-19 (page 65): Sanders M: *Mosby's paramedic textbook revised,* ed 2, St Louis, 2001, Mosby.

Figure 3-20 (page 66): Sanders M: *Mosby's paramedic textbook revised,* ed 2, St Louis, 2001, Mosby.

Figure 3-21 (page 67): Aehlert B: *ECGs made easy,* ed 2, St Louis, 2002, Mosby.

Figure 3-22 (page 68): Sanders M: *Mosby's paramedic textbook revised,* ed 2, St Louis, 2001, Mosby.

Figure 4-1 (page 73): Shade B et al: *Mosby's EMT-intermediate textbook,* ed 2, St Louis, 2002, Mosby.

Figure 4-2 (page 78): Shade B et al: *Mosby's EMT-intermediate textbook,* ed 2, St Louis, 2002, Mosby.

Figure 5-1 (page 85): Shade B et al: *Mosby's EMT-intermediate textbook,* ed 2, St Louis, 2002, Mosby.

Figure 5-2 (page 91): Sanders M: *Mosby's paramedic textbook revised,* ed 2, St Louis, 2001, Mosby.

Figure 6-1 (page 105): Sanders M: *Mosby's paramedic textbook revised,* ed 2, St Louis, 2001, Mosby.

Figure 6-2 (page 107): Sanders M: *Mosby's paramedic textbook revised,* ed 2, St Louis, 2001, Mosby.

Figure 6-3 (page 109): Sanders M: *Mosby's paramedic textbook revised,* ed 2, St Louis, 2001, Mosby.

Figure 6-4 (page 111): Sanders M: *Mosby's paramedic textbook revised,* ed 2, St Louis, 2001, Mosby.

Figure 7-1 (page 116): Thibodeau G, Patton K: *Anthony's textbook of anatomy and physiology,* ed 16, St Louis, 1999, Mosby.

Figure 7-2 (page 118): Thibodeau G, Patton K: *Anthony's textbook of anatomy and physiology,* ed 16, St Louis, 1999, Mosby.

Figure 7-3 (page 119): Thibodeau G, Patton K: *Anthony's textbook of anatomy and physiology,* ed 16, St Louis, 1999, Mosby.

Figure 7-4 (page 121): Sanders M: *Mosby's paramedic textbook revised,* ed 2, St Louis, 2001, Mosby.

Figure 7-5 (page 123): Sanders M: *Mosby's paramedic textbook revised,* ed 2, St Louis, 2001, Mosby.

Figure 7-6 (page 125): Sanders M: *Mosby's paramedic textbook revised,* ed 2, St Louis, 2001, Mosby.

Figure 7-7 (page 127): Shade B et al: *Mosby's EMT-intermediate textbook,* ed 2, St Louis, 2002, Mosby.

Figure 7-8, A-B (page 132): Thibodeau G, Patton K: *Anthony's textbook of anatomy and physiology,* ed 16, St Louis, 1999, Mosby.

Figure 7-8, C-D (page 133): C, Aehlert B: *ECGs made easy,* ed 2, St Louis, 2002, Mosby. **D,** Huszar R: *Basic dysrhythmias interpretation and management,* ed 3, St Louis, 2002, Mosby.

Unnumbered Figures

Pages 16, 47, 48: Sanders M: *Mosby's paramedic textbook revised,* ed 2, St Louis, 2001, Mosby.

Index

Page references followed by "f" indicate figures, "t" indicate tables,
and "b" indicate boxes.

R

Rectal medication administration, 89-90
Red blood cells
  low count, 4
  and oxygen saturation, 106
Reflexes, and respiration, 3
Repolarization
  definition of, 6
  and electrocardiography (ECG), 36-68
Respiratory distress
  case study, 139, 148-149
  chronic obstructive pulmonary disease (COPD), 115-126
  and nasotracheal intubation, 20-24
  nebulizers, 85-86, 87b-88b
  "on the scene" procedures, 24, 28
  orotracheal intubation for, 10
Respiratory rate, 160
Respiratory system
  anatomical diagram of, 3f
  anatomy and physiology of, 1-6
  emergencies, 115-134
  major functions of, 2-4
Rhonchi, 117, 125
  definition of, 114, 160
Rhythms, common ECG, 50f-68f
Right atria, definition and illustration of, 4, 5f, 6
Right ventricles, function and illustration of, 4, 5f, 6
R-R intervals, 50f-68f

S

Sellick's maneuver; *See* cricoid pressure
Severe respiratory distress; *See* respiratory distress
Sharps containers, needed before intubation, 14
Sinoatrial (SA) nodes
  definition of, 2, 160
  function of, 6

Sinoatrial nodes—cont'd
  generating electrical impulses, 36-37
Sinus bradycardia, electrocardiogram of, 51f
Sinus tachycardia, electrocardiogram of, 52f
Sodium bicarbonate, 100
Sodium chloride, 74
ST segment, 160
Stable angina, 129-130
Status asthmaticus, 114, 160
Status epilepticus, 84, 94, 160
Sternal intraosseous (IO) infusion, 78
Stylet, definition of, 8, 160
Suctioning
  endotracheal, 25-28
  tracheal, 10-11
Superior venae cavae, function and illustration of, 4, 5f, 6
Surfactant, 160
Sweating; *See* diaphoresis
Sympathetic nervous system, 160
Sympatholytic substance, 160
Sympathomimetic substance, 84, 97, 160
Sync, 40
Synchronized cardioversion
  definition of, 36, 161
  using ECG for, 38
Syncope, 161
Systemic circulation, 5f

T

Tachycardia
  ECG illustrations of, 54f, 59f, 65f
  during electrocardiography (ECG), 39
Tension pneumothorax, 30, 32b, 33
Thrombophlebitis
  definition of, 70, 161
  with intravenous (IV) cannulation, 71